Saw Palmetto
for Men & Women

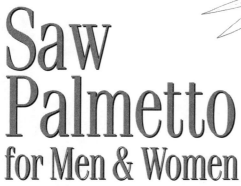

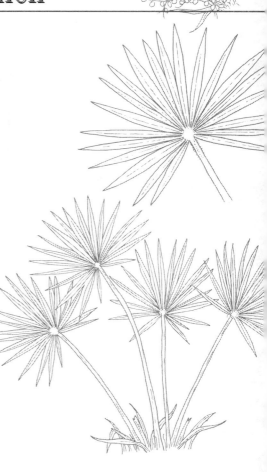

Saw Palmetto
for Men & Women

Herbal Healing for the

- **Prostate**
- **Urinary Tract**
- **Immune System and More**

David Winston,
Herbalist AHG

STOREY BOOKS

Schoolhouse Road
Pownal, Vermont 05261

The mission of Storey Communications is to serve our customers
by publishing practical information that encourages
personal independence in harmony with the environment.

Edited by Deborah Balmuth and Nancy Ringer
Cover design by Meredith Maker
Cover art production and text design by Betty Kodela
Text production by Mary Minella and Jennifer Jepson Smith
Illustrations by Sarah Brill, except on pages 1, 23, 53, 63, 65 (bottom), and 74 by
    Beverly Duncan; page 64 by Mallory Lake
Indexed by Barbara Hagerty

Printed in the United States by R.R. Donnelley
10 9 8 7 6 5 4 3 2 1

Library of Congress Cataloging-in-Publication Data

Winston, David.
    Saw palmetto for men & women / David Winston.
        p.   cm. — (A medicinal herb guide)
    Includes bibliographical references and index.
    ISBN 1-58017-206-7 (pbk. : alk. paper)
    1. Saw palmetto—Therapeutic use.   2. Benign prostatic hyperplasia—
Alternative treatment.   I. Title.   II. Title: Saw palmetto for men and women.
    III. Series.
RM666.S28W54   1999
615'.3245—dc21   99-37566
                                                                            CIP

DEDICATION

To the herbs, roots, flowers, and berries
that have taught me so much.
To my teachers, patients, students, and colleagues
who have helped me gain my knowledge and experience.
And to Carol
for her love, help, encouragement, and support.
I give thanks, Wado.

CONTENTS

ACKNOWLEDGMENTS

I would like to thank Phyllis Herman for initiating this project and helping me to overcome my writing phobia.

Marlin Huffman of Plantation Botanicals was very helpful and generous with information on saw palmetto, as was Chris Ellithorpe.

I appreciate my fellow herbalists and other practitioners who took the time to contribute case histories and their personal experiences with saw palmetto.

I also thank my office staff for endless retyping and attempting to translate my handwriting.

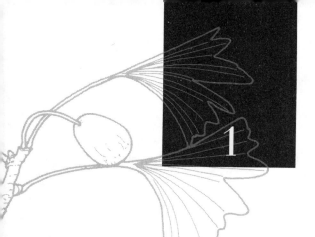

WHY CONSIDER HERBAL MEDICINE?

Welcome to the Herbal Renaissance! Having finally left the "Herbal Dark Ages," the United States is beginning to catch up to the rest of the world. From the 1920s through the late 1960s, except for a few ethnic communities (African-American, Native American, Chinese, and Hispanic), herbal medicine ceased to exist within the dominant culture in this country.

As we enter the twenty-first century, the popularity of herbs grows daily. A *Prevention/NBC Today* Saturday survey of March 1, 1997, found that one in three adults have used medicinal herbs. Market sales of herbal products were close to $3 billion in 1997, and according to the *Prevention/NBC Today* survey, most consumers who use them consider them safe, effective, and reasonably priced. In 1996, 1997, and 1998, saw palmetto was one of the top-ten best-selling herbs in the United States, with 1997 sales of $18.4 million and sales for the first half of 1998 increasing 138%. While popular literature has focused on saw palmetto's use in addressing prostate problems, it can used effectively and safely by both men and women to prevent disease and optimize their health. Why consider using saw palmetto? What can herbs do for you? Let me offer my perspective on the unique benefits of herbal medicine and what it has to offer you and our health care system.

A HEALTH-CARE SYSTEM IN CRISIS

We like to think the medicine practiced in our hospitals and medical centers is the best in the world. It is the most expensive, to be sure, and the most technologically advanced, absolutely. But these two factors are not necessarily the standards that usually define something as being "the best." According to a report published by Rob McCaleb of the Herb Research Foundation in 1997, as a percentage of gross national product, Americans pay twice as much as Europeans and three times as much as the Japanese for health care costs, yet we lag behind both groups in terms of measurable health statistics such as longevity, infant mortality, cancer, and heart disease rates.

Our health care system is in a crisis. Expenses continue to rise; cost control measures reduce the quality of care; government regulation and the resulting mountain of paperwork rarely "fix" the problems. In fact, greater regulation may often make things more complex. According to a report on National Public Radio, the average HMO physician spends just seven minutes per patient. This financial time constraint may help the bottom line, but it is damaging to the patient and the physician. There is no "healing" relationship between doctor and patient, no sense of the trust and personal connection that are so necessary for medicine to be effective.

Iatrogenic (doctor- or drug-induced) disease is another major concern. Patients are wary of health problems that develop as a result of the innate dangers of prescription medication, cross-drug interactions, and wrongly prescribed medication. Patients' fears concerning the use of pharmaceuticals are well founded: adverse reactions to medications are the fifth leading cause of death in the United States. A report in the April 1998 issue of the *Journal of the American Medical Association* estimated that in 1994, 2,216,000 hospital patients had serious adverse drug reactions, and 106,000 people died as a result of drug reactions from improperly prescribed medications. The authors of the study suggested that these figures may have actually underreported the number of such events. Awareness of these dangers associated with our current medical model and hospital care has led to increased distrust and dissatisfaction with the system. As a result, lay people are practicing greater self-care and the potentially dangerous practice of self-diagnosis.

THE GROWING INTEREST IN HERBAL MEDICINE

Ten years ago I worked as a consultant to a dozen medical practitioners. Now, I regularly consult with more than 120 physicians. Why? In part, it is because I am better known The more important reason is that most physicians know very little about herbal medicine, and their patients, in large numbers, are now taking herbal products. In fact, a recent consumer research survey released in 1998 reported that 42 percent of the people polled used some form of alternative medicine. The survey also noted that 75 percent of the people said they would be likely to use herbal medicine, and 74 percent of those reporting the use of alternative medical said they used it along with conventional health care. Of those people, 61 percent reported that their physicians were aware of these complementary treatments.

Initially, many physicians want information. Is this herb safe? Does it have possible adverse reactions? Will it interact with the patient's medication? Could it actually be beneficial? As their knowledge grows they often become excited to find that this "alternative" can offer patients an effective treatment that costs less, often has few or no side effects, and allows patients greater participation in their own health care.

Herbal medicine is integrated into the medical systems of many countries throughout the world. In Japan, Germany, China, India, Italy, Austria, France, and Sweden, a visit to a doctor is likely to produce an herbal prescription instead of one for a pharmaceutical drug. According to an article in *The New York Times*, prescriptions for St.-John's-wort for depression outnumber prescriptions for Prozac by 4 to 1 in Germany. We are an exception in this country, and our medical system is the poorer due to this fact. For many conditions such as osteoarthritis, premenstrual syndrome, menopausal symptoms, skin conditions such as eczema or psoriasis, attention deficit disorder, and poor peripheral circulation, properly prescribed herbs can be a first choice in intelligent treatment. In other more serious conditions, herbs can be valuable adjuncts to orthodox treatment. Practitioners with whom I consult regularly incorporate herbal protocols into treatments for atheriosclerosis, degenerative kidney disease, hepatitis B and C, arthralgias, and many other diseases.

A good example of this "best of both worlds" therapy happened a few years ago.

A friend's wife came down with bacterial meningitis. She was rushed to the hospital and given intravenous antibiotics, and she recovered from this dangerous life-threatening disease. (In this type of acute health emergency, you want the great benefits of Western medicine, not herbs, bodywork, or relaxation techniques.) Upon her release from the hospital, she was still experiencing serious problems from her disease. She had severe visual, auditory, and tactile disturbances. She had trouble seeing, hearing, talking, and remembering. Her physician hoped that these cognitive disturbances would resolve within six months, but he could offer no treatment. An herbal protocol was started, and within two weeks the majority of these problems were gone. By four weeks later, she was fully recovered. Without any doubts, I attribute this quick recovery to the effective combination of Western treatment and herbal follow-up care.

This case of herbs complementing technology is not an isolated incident — I have had similar experiences with other conditions. For example, although best treated initially by Western medicine, traumatic head injuries have responded well to adjunctive herbal therapies, as have various cancers, heart disease, and autoimmune disorders such as lupus, ankylosing spondylitis, and scleroderma.

COMMON MISCONCEPTIONS ABOUT HERBS

Because Americans have little experience with herbs, we are poorly educated about their benefits and dangers. It is vital that as we start to use herbs we educate ourselves not only to the benefits they can provide but to their drawbacks and possible dangers. I believe the average American has two major misconceptions about herbs.

Natural Does Not Mean Safe

Many people believe that because herbs are "natural" they are therefore safe and nontoxic. This can be a dangerous belief, as many natural plants (foxglove, belladonna, poison hemlock, and even rhubarb leaf) are extremely toxic. Strong herbal medicines such as poke root *(Phytolacca americana)*, blue flag *(Iris versicolor)*, bloodroot *(Sanguinaria canadensis)*, and even the common spice nutmeg can produce dangerous effects if they are used incorrectly or in too great amounts.

In Cherokee (Ani Yunwiya) medicine, one of the oldest and most diverse of Native American medical systems, plants are divided into three categories depending on how they affect people. The first category is the food herbs. These are generally safe, nontoxic remedies that can be taken in substantial quantities for continuous periods of time. These herbs are appropriate for self-treatment of mild, self-limiting diseases. They generally act as tonic remedies to enhance nutrition and strengthen organ function. Herbs such as dandelion leaf and root *(Taraxacum officinale)*, hawthorn berry *(Crataegus monogyna)*, red clover *(Trifolium pratense)*, chamomile *(Matricaria recutita)*, nettles *(Urtica dioica)*, peppermint *(Mentha piperita)*, garlic *(Allium sativum)*, ginger *(Zingaberis officinalis)*, shiitake mushroom *(Lentinula edodes)*, and saw palmetto *(Serenoa repens)* fit into this category.

The second category is the medicinal herbs. These are stronger-acting plants that are used for specific problems and for specific periods of time, then discontinued. These medicines are not tonic herbs, and they have a greater potential for adverse reactions. A few herbs in this category include the overutilized and endangered goldenseal *(Hydrastis canadensis)* as well as black cohosh *(Cimicifuga racemosa)*, eucalyptus *(Eucalyptus globulus)*, ma huang *(Ephedra sinensis)*, blue cohosh root *(Caulophyllum thalictroides)*, chaparral *(Larrea* spp.), horse chestnut *(Aesculus hippocastanum)*, and kava *(Piper methysticum)*.

The third group of herbs is the poisons. These plants have a strong potential for toxic reactions and should never be taken without a recommendation and supervision from a medical herbalist — often certified as Herbalist AHG (peer-reviewed professional member of the American Herbalists Guild) or MNIMH (member of the British National Institute of Medical Herbalists) — or a physician. Self-experimentation with these plants is dangerous and may lead to severe injury or even death. Poisonous plants include gelsemium *(Gelsemium sempirvirens)*, dogbane *(Apocynum cannabinum)*, aconite *(Aconitum* spp.), lily of the valley *(Convallaria majalis)*, and henbane *(Hyoscyamus niger)* as well as the previously mentioned toxic plants (foxglove, poison hemlock, belladonna, poke root, bloodroot). An important reminder comes from the Hippocratic Oath, "First Do No Harm." This warning is appropriate for any practitioner or the person who undertakes self-treatment. Potentially toxic herbs should be used only by practitioners who have been trained to use them and who understand the toxicology, pharmacology, and antidotes for such powerful medicines.

More Is Not Necessarily Better

Along with the false belief that natural equals safe, another common misconception is that if a little bit is good, more must be better. We see this milligram escalation in television commercials.

CHEROKEE MEDICINE PLANT CLASSIFICATIONS

Food Herbs: Safe, nontoxic herbs that can be taken in substantial quantities for continuous periods of time. Any substance can possibly cause an allergic reaction or idiosyncratic response. The first time you eat a new food or take a new herb, the dosage should be small and then gradually built up to the normal dosage.

Medicine Herbs: Useful for specific problems; should be taken for specified periods of time only.

Poison Herbs: Can cause toxic or fatal reactions; should not be taken without a recommendation and supervision from a medical herbalist or physician.

One company has a 500-milligram aspirin, the next a 750-milligram aspirin, and a third claims superiority by having a 1000-milligram tablet. The companies are suggesting that more equal better, but with herbs this concept does not necessarily apply. Many stronger herbs have one effect in small doses but have an opposite effect in larger doses. A good example is the wild ginger root *(Asarum canadensis)*. Small amounts of the tea (2 to 4 ounces, two or three times per day) will relieve nausea, vomiting, and gas. Larger amounts can have the opposite effect and can cause intense nausea, vomiting, and gas. A second example is the potentially toxic herb bloodroot *(Sanguinaria canadensis)*. Very small amounts of the tincture are used by practitioners to stop dry, persistent coughs. Take just a fraction too much, and this acrid root will cause the irritated cough to worsen dramatically. There is no substitute for intelligent use of herbs based on traditional use, modern research, and clinical experience.

HERBAL TREATMENT
NEEDS TO BE INDIVIDUALIZED

Another problem in the growing herbal market is the increasing commercialization of herbs. Many consumers get their information from companies selling herbs; unfortunately, these companies are not an unbiased source. Vitamin companies are now vitamin and herb companies. Pharmaceutical giants, seeing a growing market, are now producing herbal products. Many herbal formulas that are widely marketed include a dizzying range of herbs, the theory being that if you include a wide array of herbs in the formula, maybe something will work. This is bad herbal medicine.

A good herbalist treats people, not diseases. Ten patients diagnosed with rheumatoid arthritis would get ten different protocols based on their unique constitutions and symptom pictures. Some parts of the treatments may overlap, but Chris Smith, who is 72 years old, chronically constipated, has impaired circulation, and suffers from insomnia in addition to rheumatoid arthritis, presents a very different picture than does Angela Jones, who is 32 years old, has terrible premenstrual and menstrual problems, hyperchlorhydria (excess stomach acid), and migraine headaches as well as rheumatoid arthritis. A well-done herbal protocol will use differential diagnosis and energetics to create a specific treatment for each person.

Diagnostic Techniques

Differential diagnosis — the identification of the patient's illness as distinguished from illnesses with similar features — is used in Western medicine as well as Chinese, Ayurvedic, Cherokee, and most other systems of medicine. The diagnostic techniques differ widely but give the practitioner useful clues to what is actually happening in the patient. In Western medicine, blood and urine tests, computed tomography, magnetic resonance imaging, and biopsies as well as physical diagnostic techniques are commonly used. In Eastern medicine, analysis of the tongue, pulse, and face is used, along with general observation, stool and urine analysis, plus five-elements typing. In Western medicine, diagnosis confirms or disproves the gross pathologic changes of disease. In most indigenous systems of medicine, diagnostic techniques show patterns of disharmony. In the later stages of disease, this will reflect the same gross pathologic conditions shown by Western diagnosis. But at its best, traditional diagnosis shows imbalances of subtle energies that occur months or years before overt pathologic changes occur.

I am reminded of a wonderful example. In the motion picture *The Last Emperor,* when the emperor was still a young child, he used his potty-seat. His physician examined his fresh stool and immediately announced "no meat, no tofu." What he saw were signs of excess heat and dryness in the stool. Instead of ignoring a minor imbalance, he changed the young emperor's diet to prevent greater disharmony and possible future illness.

The Chinese concept of energetics states that each medicine has a temperament or nature: it is heating or cooling, moistening or drying, condensing or dispersing. The same can be said of diseases. Fevers and inflammations are usually a sign of excess heat; chronic low-grade diarrhea is most often a sign of dampness; dry eyes, a dry mouth, a dry cough, and sticky sputum are signs of excess dryness. Herbs are used accordingly to balance the disharmonies: cooling and moistening herbs for hot dry conditions; warming, drying, and fragrant herbs for cold damp conditions. I hope this very simple example will help the reader gain a basic idea of the concept of energetics.

The "one size fits all" mentality found throughout the popular herbal literature suggests that a generic formula in the store — let's call it "headache herbs" — is effective for all headaches and for all people. This is ridiculous, as there are many types of headaches, and even with the same type (such as migraines or cluster headache), each person should still be given an individual formula.

First, we need to understand why the person is experiencing headaches. Are they stress related? Does the person have muscle spasms of the neck and scalp muscles, temporomandibular joint (TMJ) dysfunction, or subluxation of the cervical vertebrae? Could the problem be related to environmental allergies causing sinus pressure? Could it be caused by food allergies or trigger foods (wheat, chocolate, coffee, aspartame, etc.)? Are chronic constipation, hypertension, or liver problems present? Is the person in great physical, mental, or spiritual distress? To be effective, we need to understand the underlying cause and the energetics of the condition. Then we can appropriately recommend herbs, dietary changes, stress reduction techniques, a visit to a doctor, or whatever is really needed.

Willow bark, which is an anodyne (painkiller), may help mild headache pain but doesn't address the underlying constitutional issues. Kava, an antianxiety agent and antispasmodic, is useful for muscle spasms and anxiety-driven head pain but is ineffective for sinus headaches. Feverfew, a bitter anti-inflammatory, helps vasodilative migraines but does little for vasoconstrictive headaches or those caused by TMJ dysfunction.

Appreciating the Complexity of Herbs

In this age of advertising and fast-moving media images, herbs are reduced to their lowest common denominator. Instead of learning about their personality, we accept sound bite images. So St.-John's-wort is now touted as the "depression herb," milk thistle as the "liver herb," and bilberry as the "eye herb." To quote my friend Mark Blumenthal, president of the American Botanical Council, "If the industry could find an organ for grape seed extract, its sales would rise spectacularly. It's a flavonoid in search of an organ." In the magazines, saw palmetto is frequently featured as the "prostate herb." In this book, I hope to show you that saw palmetto is not only a useful herb for prostate problems but clearly has benefits for the male and female reproductive systems and for immune function, the lungs, the urinary tract, and the endocrine glands.

I hope the reader will profit from this, my first book. Together we will continue to gain knowledge and experience in using herbs. After 31 years of learning, practicing, and teaching about herbs, I feel comfortable calling myself an "advanced" beginner. This is only partially in jest, as the world of herbal medicine is vast, and it truly is a lifelong study. I've been fortunate enough to be trained in Cherokee, Chinese, and eclectic/Western traditions, and I believe my synthesis of these systems is especially useful for the herbal neophyte as well as for herbalists who have not been trained in a specific system of herbal medicine.

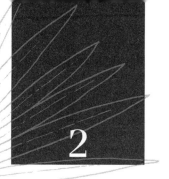

AN INTRODUCTION TO SAW PALMETTO
Getting to Know the Plant

Native to the coastal regions of the Southeastern United States, saw palmetto is a small creeping shrub or shrubby tree, 4 to 8 feet tall, that grows in dense colonies called palmetto scrubs in coastal South Carolina, southern Georgia, Florida, southern Alabama, and southeastern Louisiana. This hardy, almost weedy plant grows in sandy soils and thin woods, and is most plentiful near the coast. It will tolerate poor, even saline soil and will regenerate quickly after a fire. In the 1870s one continuous grove of saw palmetto in Florida was noted to stretch over 100 miles from Mosquito Inlet to Jupiter Inlet.

The name "saw" palmetto comes from the sharp-edged fan-shaped leaves. The bladelike serrated edges create nearly impenetrable thickets. The leaves are palmate (fan-shaped) and are divided into 18 to 24 lance-shaped leaflets. The leaves range in color from blue-green to yellow-green to an almost silvery white. The aromatic flowers are an ivory-white color and are found in large clusters, May through July.

The "berries" of saw palmetto are botanically known as drupes. They are found on the branching spadices, which form large pendulous panicles, or clusters, of fruit 18 to 24 inches long and weighing 6 to 8 pounds. As they ripen in September through

Overview of Saw Palmetto

- **Botanical name:** *Serenoa repens*, of the Palmae Family. Saw palmetto was named after the noted botanist Professor Sereno Watson of Harvard University.
- **Common names:** Fan palm, dwarf palmetto, Sägepalmenfrüchte (German), sabal vruchten (Dutch), fruits de sabal (French).
- **Part used:** Berry.
- **Taste:** Sweet, acrid.
- **Energy:** Warm, moist.
- **Western classification:** Adaptogen, antiandrogenic, anti-inflammatory, diuretic, expectorant, immune amphoteric, urinary antiseptic, demulcent.
- **Chinese classification:** Yin tonic to the Lungs, Spleen, and Kidney; Qi tonic.
- **Primary modern uses:** Anorexia, benign prostatic hyperplasia, irritable bladder, abacterial prostatitis with a mucus discharge, immune deficiency, laryngitis, dysuria, female hirsutism, cystitis with irritation and tenesmic pain, ovarian and uterine pain, polycystic ovary disease, chronic bronchial irritation, mild asthmatic chronic obstructive pulmonary disease, pelvic congestion, chronic irritative cough.
- **Possible uses:** Male pattern baldness, prostate cancer, male and female infertility, cystic acne, "male menopause."
- **Contraindications:** Damp spleen conditions: chronic flatulence, low-grade diarrhea, abdominal bloating, borborygmus.
- **Side effects:** Occasional mild nausea and gastric upset, rarely headache, possibly diarrhea if large quantities are used.
- **Drug interactions:** According to the German Komission E, none known.
- **Potential problems:** There is concern that saw palmetto might hide elevated prostate specific antigen (PSA) levels, thus preventing early detection of prostatic cancer. Recent studies from France, published in *The Prostate* in 1996, show no change in PSA levels even after men have taken saw palmetto for one year. According to studies done by Italian phytopharmaceutical manufacturer Indena S. P. A., saw palmetto extracts are devoid of any mutagenic or teratogenic effects.

December, the olive-sized (½ to 1 inch) fruits turn a dark purplish black color with a oily sheen and a strong odor. The odor has been compared to that of overripe cheese. Inside the juicy flesh is a single hard, white, oily seed. The dried "berry" should be in its whole form; it will be shriveled, have a dark purplish black color, and retain its characteristic odor. In addition, good-quality berries should be free of any mold, dust, insect damage, and pathogenic bacteria.

Wild plants tend to bear large quantities of fruit every other year. With the increasing demand for this herb, there have been occasional shortages of saw palmetto during the years when the shrubby trees produce a smaller crop.

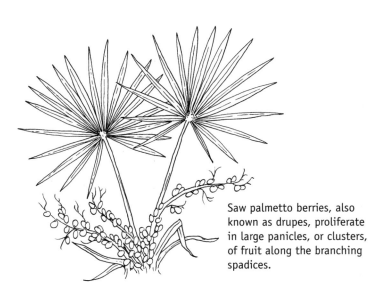

Saw palmetto berries, also known as drupes, proliferate in large panicles, or clusters, of fruit along the branching spadices.

CHEMISTRY OF THE BERRIES

Anyone who has ever handled these fruits is aware of their oily nature. They contain approximately 1.5 percent of a strong-smelling pungent oil. Sixty-three to sixty-five percent of this oil consists of free fatty acids such as capric, caproic, caprylic, lauric, linoleic, linolenic, oleic, myristic, palmitic, and stearic acids. The remaining oil content is made of ethyl esters of these fatty acids and sterols such as beta-sitosterol, stigmasterol, lupeol, and campesterol. Other active constituents include diterpenes, such as geranylgeraniol and phytol; triterpenes, such as cycloartenal and lupeol; sesquiterpenes, such as farnesol; and high-molecular-weight alcohols, including N-docosanol, N-octacosanol, N-tricosanol, and hexacosanol.

Various carotenoids, tannins, and invert sugars (28 percent), and a small quantity of volatile oils (vanillic acid, vanillin, and ferulic acid), are also found in the berries. Professor Wagner, a world-renowned pharmacognocist at the University of Munchen in Germany, has shown that the immune-enhancing constituents of the herb are water soluble. Teas or capsules of saw palmetto contain high-molecular-weight polysaccharides known as S1, S2, S3, and S4, which contain the sugars glucose, galactose, mannose, fucose, arabinose, rhamnose, and glucuronic acid. These immune-stimulating compounds are largely absent from standardized gel caps and tinctures with a high alcohol content (more than 40 percent).

The list on the following page, compiled from the USDA phytochemical database of James A. Duke, Ph.D., details some of the chemical compounds found in the saw palmetto fruit and their known activities. As with most herbal medicines, the sum of the parts — the synergy of the plant's chemistry — has greater activity than any single chemical entity contained in the plant.

CHEMICAL COMPOUNDS FOUND IN SAW PALMETTO FRUIT

CHEMICAL	USEFUL PROPERTIES
Anthranilic acid	Anti-inflammatory, antiarthritic
Apigenin	Anti-inflammatory, antiestrogenic, antioxidant, antitumor, antihistamine, antispasmodic
Beta-sitosterol D-glucoside	Antitumor, antispasmodic
Campesterol	Anti-inflammatory
Cycloartenol	Bactericide, hypocholesterolemic
Farnesol	Antitumor, antispasmodic, sedative
Ferulic acid	Analgesic, anti-inflammatory, antiestrogenic, antispasmodic, antimutagenic, bactericide, immunostimulant
Kaempferol	Antihistamine, anti-inflammatory, antioxidant, antitumor, factor inhibitor
Mannitol	Anti-inflammatory, antimutagenic, antioxidant
Stigmasterol	Anti-inflammatory, antitumor, cholesterol-lowering activity
Syringaldehyde	Anti-inflammatory, cancer preventive
Vanillic acid	Anti-inflammatory, antioxidant, bactericide, cancer preventive

COLLECTING AND PREPARING SAW PALMETTO

Because of the great abundance of wild saw palmetto, most of it was harvested in the wild until the recent surge in demand for it. Gathering one's own saw palmetto in the wild can be a challenging task. Tough clothing and gloves are necessary for protection from cutting by the sharp leaves; at the same time, heavy clothing is uncomfortable because of the warm and humid climate.

Poisonous snakes such as diamondback rattlesnakes are a very real danger to saw palmetto harvesters, as are spiders and scorpions.

Florida has recently struggled with legal issues concerning *Serenoa*. As demand has risen, so has illegal gathering of the berries from private lands and parklands. Recent legislative efforts have been made to require processors to record the source of the berries they purchase. Fines and confiscation of black-market (stolen) saw palmetto are possible penalties if these laws are eventually adopted.

A common practice of wildcrafters is to shake the shrubs so that the fruit falls into a wide-mouthed basket, pail, or net. Another method of collecting the fruit is to clip the fruit stem (spadice) with pruning shears and catch the panicles of fruit as they fall. Estimates from the University of Florida suggest that less than 3 percent of the total berry crop is gathered. Thus, this plant is in little danger of overharvesting and can be considered a renewable resource.

Growing Saw Palmetto

There has been increased "cultivation" of saw palmetto, mostly to make it easier to harvest. Over 250,000 acres of saw palmetto plantations are semicultivated. These "plantations" are burned yearly after harvest to reduce undergrowth, make harvesting easier, and stimulate the next year's production. The burning process is called a controlled burn. The fire is kept small and relatively cool to protect the heart of the palm from damage.

In addition to yearly burning, beehives are kept in the palmetto groves to insure pollination, which improves the crop's yield. One company, Plantation Botanicals, is experimenting with true cultivation of *Serenoa* in Guatemala, but because of the easy availability of wild material, actual farm cultivation is not currently financially feasible.

When saw palmetto berries were taken from the wild there was little impact on the environment because harvesters mainly gathered easily accessible berries and avoided dense thickets.

Large-scale plantations may be problematic in several ways. First, yearly burning adds to air pollution, creating increased carbon monoxide and particulates, and possibly contributing to global warming. The second problem has to do with animal habitat. Much of the land now considered to be "plantations" was previously left alone, infested with the "useless weed" saw palmetto. With little human disturbance, this land provided refuge for the endangered Everglades panther and black bears. Yearly burning and greater human encroachment may further the possibility of extinction of these threatened species.

Processing and Drying the Berries

The picked berries are partially dried on trays by sunlight or artificial heat until they reach the consistency of a prune. The berries are then sorted, and the final drying is done with low-temperature artificial heat until they are fully dried. Berries that are sun-dried or gathered farther inland (more than 4 or 5 miles from the coast) are considered to be of inferior quality.

Recent large-scale production has required companies to upgrade their drying technology. Thermostatically controlled kilns are now used by large suppliers to dry these berries, and it takes up to 5 days to fully dry them. When the berries are fully dried to a moisture content of 7.5 percent, they are supposedly stable and medicinally active. With the constant admonishments from eclectic health care practitioners that only the semi-fresh berries are truly active, it would be interesting to see comparative studies on the activity of medicines made with one versus the other.

The dried berries have a shelf-life of approximately one year when stored in an airtight glass or ceramic container in a dark, dry environment. (Sunlight, humidity, and heat can all degrade the activity of the herb.) Any berries with mold on them should be discarded.

SAW PALMETTO PREPARATIONS

Making your own herbal preparations can be a challenging but fascinating process. Herbal pharmacy can be as simple as making a cup of tea can or much more complex, as in making a tincture. Some processes can easily be done at home with little equipment other than standard kitchenware. Producing your own teas, salves, vinegar, honey extracts, and cough syrups and filling capsules can save you money and be a wonderful part of the healing process. Making your own alcohol-water extracts (tinctures), solid extracts, and glycerites is a much more exacting process. Unless you are willing to take the time to learn the necessary procedures, purchasing well-made products may prove a better choice.

Tea

Tea formulations made from the dried berries are probably the least effective way of taking saw palmetto for prostate or polycystic ovary problems because the fatty sterols are not water soluble. However, saw palmetto tea is effective for strengthening the immune system and as a tonic to the Lung Qi. The greatest problem with saw palmetto berry tea is the rather awful taste.

To make a tea of saw palmetto, combine 2 teaspoons of the dried berry in a saucepan with 24 ounces of water. Slowly simmer for 1 hour until the liquid is reduced by half. The dose is 4 ounces of the tea three times per day. Adding a sweetener such as honey will do little to improve the taste.

Capsules

The effectiveness of saw palmetto capsules containing the ground herb depends on the quality of the ground berries. Older berries lose their activity and effectiveness. A good-quality product has a strong odor and a pungent aromatic taste. The dosage is 2 or 3 capsules, three times per day (1 to 2 grams per day). OO (15-grain) capsules are available in most health food stores as well as many pharmacies. It is a simple but tedious process to fill your own capsules by hand. Small capsule-filling devices are available and can speed up the process considerably.

Tincture

To make a tincture, which is a hydroalcoholic (water and alcohol) extract, use 1 part semifresh berries for every 3 parts of solution made up of 70 percent ethyl alcohol and 30 percent water. The dosage is 3 to 4 milliliters (60 to 80 drops), three to four times a day. Eclectic practitioners believed that the best preparation of *Serenoa* is made with the fresh ripe berries. The extract should have a strong, ethereal, aromatic flavor and will precipitate when it is mixed in large amounts with water. In small amounts it produces an opalescent mixture. If it is rubbed between the fingers, a greasy sensation occurs, and the pronounced aroma of the berries is quite obvious.

Homeopathic Mother Tincture

In homeopathy (see the discussion of this type of medicine in chapter 4), a dilute alcohol/water extract is used as a base for preparing other medicines. This preparation is called the mother tincture and it is made in a 1:10 dilution with the fresh ripe berries. The directions for its manufacture in the *Homeopathic Pharmacopoeia* are as follows:
  • *Sabal serrulata,* moist magma containing plant solids (100 grams) — the fresh ground plant
  • Plant moisture 500 cubic centimeters (600 grams) — the liquid found in the plant
  • Strong alcohol 95 percent (537 cubic centimeters)
  This makes 1000 cubic centimeters of tincture. Dosage of the mother tincture is 1 to 60 drops. Homeopathic medicine also uses this tincture in dilutions of 3 times and higher.

Standardized Gel Caps

This last category of saw palmetto product is a recent introduction to the world of herbs. Standardized products are manufactured to contain specific amounts of phytochemicals that the producers believe may be active constituents or that act as marker chemicals (a specific, easy-to-test-for component of the herb). The idea is that every capsule contains the exact same measure of the active substance. There are both pros and cons concerning this type of product and we will discuss them further in chapter 5.

While most people believe that all standardized products are the same, different manufacturers use very different processing procedures, most of which are unique to their particular companies. The issue of phytoequivalence (whether two different standardized products are really the same) is a valid concern. According to research done in France, the chemical composition and especially the activity of different standardized extracts can vary widely.

Saw palmetto gel caps are manufactured by two basic processes. The first uses hexane and the dried, powdered fruit. This is done in an inert gas atmosphere with antioxidants such as ascorbic palmitate. The second technique is more expensive but involves no solvent residues. Carbon dioxide is used in supercritical extraction (a high-tech method of extracting plant constituents, especially oils, under high pressure) to produce a product that is active and ready for use with no further purification.

The dosage of saw palmetto products that are standardized to 35 percent fatty acids (hexane or carbon dioxide extract) is 4 to 6 capsules per day. The recommended dosage of the 85 percent to 95 percent fatty acid product (hexane or carbon dioxide extract) is 320 milligrams per day (usually two 160-milligram capsules per day). Most studies of the herb have used this dose level, but data published by Dr. J. Braeckman in 1997 showed that there was only marginally better therapeutic activity in a 320-milligram dose than in a 160-milligram dose per day.

REGULATORY STATUS OF SAW PALMETTO IN VARIOUS COUNTRIES

Belgium: approved as prescription medication as adjunctive treatment for benign prostatic hyperplasia (enlarged prostate).

France: standardized preparations approved as ethical drugs and available through prescription only.

Germany: approved for over-the-counter use for benign prostatic hyperplasia.

Sweden: classified as a "natural product."

United Kingdom: approved for the general sales list.

United States: under DSHEA sold as a dietary supplement. *Serenoa* is also listed in the *Homeopathic Pharmacopoeia of the United States* (1979).

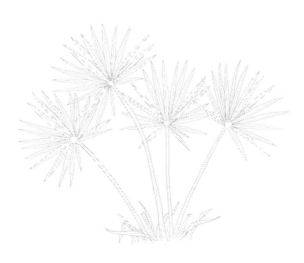

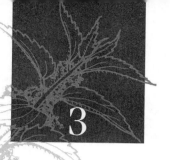

HERBALISTS'
FIRST-HAND EXPERIENCE

My introduction to saw palmetto took place in the late 1960s. Even then, when herbs were far beyond mainstream consciousness, saw palmetto was popular. In 1968, information about herbs and opportunities to study them in the United States were scarce. My early mode of learning consisted of buying all the books I could find and reading them cover to cover. Then I would identify the herb in the wild or purchase it at a health food store. Upon returning home, I would make tea and consume substantial quantities of it so I could experience the effects first hand. This technique by and large served me well, but I must admit there were some very unpleasant and foolish experiments. Senna, a strong laxative, made for a painful and extended stay in and near the bathroom. Lobelia, which in excess doses is an emetic, made me extremely nauseated and produced intense vomiting. I was cautious enough not to experiment with any of the more overtly toxic plants. I slowly gained experience to go with my growing intellectual knowledge. In the texts available at this time (Dr. Christopher's *School of Natural Healing*, Jethro Kloss's *Back to Eden*, Maude Grieve's *Modern Herbal*), saw palmetto was generally recommended for two purposes: as a reproductive tonic for men and women, and for prostatic enlargement, prostatitis, and related conditions.

DISCOVERING
SAW PALMETTO'S BENEFITS

Over the next few years, people started to inquire about what herb was good for this problem or that, and I gradually found myself telling friends, neighbors, and teachers about my experiences and the knowledge I had gained about different herbs. As I became increasingly familiar with various herbs, sometimes I found that what was in the books did not always match my practical experience. In the case of saw palmetto, I found that its effects on a normal healthy reproductive system are minimal. It is not an aphrodisiac, it will not increase the size of fully developed breasts or testicles, it doesn't shrink a swollen prostate, and it doesn't cure benign prostatic hyperplasia.

Saw palmetto is a reproductive amphoteric, and it normalizes function. If a person has a lack of libido because of exhaustion, it will nourish and strengthen your entire endocrine system, including the reproductive organs. If a person has delayed puberty or poorly developed secondary sexual characteristics, saw palmetto will help to stimulate sexual maturation and increase activity. In prostatic enlargements it will help to relieve symptoms of dysuria, nocturnal enuresis, and urinary dribbling, but by itself it will not shrink a swollen prostate.

In the years following my initial experience with saw palmetto, I began my training with my uncle in Cherokee medicine, which continued for 15 years. A short time later, I was introduced to the eclectic medical literature, and by the late 1970s I had apprenticed with a doctor of Chinese medicine in New York City. This cross-cultural training dramatically expanded my understanding of herbal practice. Different theories of medicine weren't competing: they were just different views of the world and the human organism. Each tradition has its own materia medica (materials of medicine), diagnostic techniques, and therapeutic strategies. Once you gain proficiency with these tools, it becomes clear that none of them is the "right" way to practice herbal medicine. Each system has its strengths and weaknesses, based on the underlying cultural paradigms and healing traditions. In clinical practice, it is like having three different sets of tools. When working with a patient, I determine which set of tools (Cherokee, Chinese, or Western) seems most appropriate, both for understanding the person's symptoms and for treating them. Having spent the last 31 years learning and then using the various herbs in these three systems of medicine, I find it relatively simple now to mix and match herbs on the basis of their activity, their energetic qualities, and my personal experience.

FIRST-HAND EXPERIENCE: CASE HISTORIES

The increasing knowledge of herbal medicine I was acquiring, along with university studies in sciences and Western medicine (anatomy, physiology, cellular biology, pathology, etc.) and increased clinical experience, allowed me to be creative and to find unique ways of using herbs. My clinical use of saw palmetto is no exception. It is clear to me that saw palmetto is a poorly understood herb, pigeonholed in its activity and function.

The following case histories are some of the more interesting I have dealt with over the past 30 years. The common thread, of course, is that saw palmetto was a prominent part of the therapeutic regimen. All four case descriptions are taken from actual case histories, which are much more detailed. They have been simplified for this book.

Case 1: Male Infertility

The 30-something couple who sat across from me were distraught. In their 10th year of a happy marriage, they had put off having children until they felt emotionally and financially secure. Three years earlier they had decided that the time to have a child was right. No more birth control; no more worry about an unexpected pregnancy. Lovemaking became relaxed, more fun, and wonder-fully passionate.

After a year had passed without the expected result, they started to wonder what might be wrong. They both assumed that the wife had a fertility problem, and she endured numerous tests and medical procedures. The results were unexpected. She was fine and fertile. Her husband was upset, embarrassed, and to some degree in denial that he, a strong, "virile" man, could be infertile. After a few arguments and a lot less intimacy, he finally agreed to have some tests done. The results made clear the problem. His sperm count was less than 10,000,000 sperm per milliliter of sem-inal fluid (20,000,000 sperm per milliliter or more is considered fertile), and his sperm motility was poor (less than 50 percent). His physician recommended abstinence for 3 or 4 days before his wife ovulated and suggested that he switch from tight jockey shorts to loose boxer shorts (sperm production is inhibited by temperatures over 94° to 95°F).

Another year went by, with still no results. The stress of timing sexual activity, results-oriented lovemaking, and the disappoint-ment of constant failure began to create marital problems. Beginning to search for alternatives, they tried a nutritionist (vita-min E, zinc, raw bovine testicular tissue), a hypnotist (repeat after me, your sperm is getting lively!), and homeopathy, but nothing helped. After a third year of despair, they finally came to my office, saying I was their last hope.

After a thorough interview, case history, differential diagno-sis, and diet and lifestyle history, I made the following recom-mendations: "Continue the vitamin E and zinc, discontinue the raw bovine tissue, stop smoking cigarettes and marijuana, improve the diet, get more regular sleep and exercise, AND RELAX." Chronic stress never helps normal body functions or the healing process. I suggested the following herbal tincture for-mula: saw palmetto *(Serenoa repens)* 2 parts, Chinese ginseng *(Panax ginseng)* 1 part, he shou wu *(Polygonum multiflorum)* 1 part, ashwagandha *(Withania somniferum)* 1 part, fresh milky oat

(Avena sativa) 2 parts. He took 5 milliliters of this formula three times per day. The first month he noticed he felt less anxious. The second month he stated he had increased energy with a calmer attitude. By the third month, his wife said he was much more pleasant to be with, day to day and evening to evening. The seventh month they called to tell me that they had conceived. The happy ending of this case history was a healthy baby boy and two very grateful new parents.

Case 2: Immune Deficiency with Constant Wheezing

The patient, 46 years old, said he had been sickly even as a child. Cold damp bronchitis, chest colds, sinus infections, otitis media (ear infections), pertussis (whooping cough), chronic wheezing cough, and postnasal drip had been companions for his entire life. He was tall and thin, even slightly emaciated, with a narrow chest, poor muscle tone, and pale skin. He worked as a low-level functionary in a crowded insurance office. His job was highly stressful and totally unrewarding. Every cold, flu, or other contagious illness that someone brought to work, he went home with.

The patient came to see me as a referral from his physician. Both he and his doctor were frustrated by his lack of improvement. Constant antibiotics did less and less, antihistamines made him feel miserable, and other medications showed little benefit. I was surprised at his diet, which was actually much better than I expected. The biggest problems were his overconsumption of raw vegetables (cooling energy) and his nightly bowl of ice cream. My initial suggestion included more cooked vegetables, especially foods rich in carotenoids: sweet potatoes, winter squash, carrots, apricots, watercress, pumpkin, dark green leafy vegetables, and beets. He also agreed to exclude dairy foods for 2 months to see whether that would help his postnasal drip. Differential diagnosis clearly showed he was deficient (pale, thin, weak) with deficient Lung and Spleen Qi and Deficient Xue (Blood). From a Western perspective, his immune system was impaired, his lungs were atonic, he showed signs of anemia (blood tests showed a low hemoglobin count), and while his digestion wasn't obviously impaired, he had great difficulty absorbing nutrients because of long-term antibiotic use.

His herbal protocol was more complex than for the previous patient, as we had much more to do. I suggested enteric-coated acidophilus capsules to replenish his bowel flora, along with nondairy fermented foods such as miso, unpasteurized sauerkraut, kimchee (Korean fermented cabbage), and apple cider vinegar. Herbally, warming bitters such as angelica, fenugreek, and turmeric were given to improve his ability to absorb vital nutrients. Once we had worked on improving his diet and digestion, the next part of our protocol was focused on building blood and strengthening his lungs and immune system. Although his treatment lasted over two years and his formulas were changed many times, the following tea combination was quite successful in improving his health: saw palmetto *(Serenoa repens)* 2 parts, prince ginseng *(Pseudostellaria heterophylla)* 2 parts, wu wei zi/schisandra berry *(Schisandra chinensis)* 1 part, citrus peel *(Citrus aurantium)* ½ part, huang qi/astragalus *(Astragalus membranaceus)* 1 part, ginger *(Zingiber officinale)* ½ part. The tea was made using 2 teaspoons of the mixed ground herbs to 16 ounces of water. The herbs (with the exception of ginger and citrus) were slowly decocted for 40 minutes until the liquid was reduced by half (to 8 ounces). The aromatic herbs were then added, and the combination was steeped, covered, for 1 hour. He drank two or three cups per day, taking it to work in a thermos. His first comment, as expected, concerned the taste of the tea, which he claimed had a rather odd flavor.

Within 6 weeks he had markedly reduced postnasal drip and less bronchial congestion. Although he caught a cold, he thought it was shorter than usual. After another month, he decided to reintroduce ice cream into his diet. His body's response was unequivocal: increased congestion, postnasal drip, and wheezing within 24 hours. Over the following 6 months, improvement, while gradual, was steady. The number of respiratory infections was reduced by half, he had gained weight, and blood tests revealed a normal hemoglobin count.

Another year of progress followed, with occasional downturns, but in general his life improved dramatically. He no longer lived in fear of catching every contagious illness. His occasional cold no longer inevitably wound up in his lungs. He felt more energetic, he got out more, and he took more frequent walks. His skin color looked healthier and his muscle tone improved, but he still hated his job. Well, herbs can't help everything!

Case 3: Interstitial Cystitis

One of my second-year students, a nurse practitioner who was having problems achieving positive results with her patient, brought this case discussion to class to review her assessment as well as her protocols. Her patient had one major complaint, interstitial cystitis, and two minor problems, ovarian pain during ovulation and acne during her menses. My student had already made suggestions for dietary and nutritional changes (to eliminate sugars and possible food allergens, to increase water consumption, and to take omega-3 fatty acids, zinc, and mixed carotenoids). Herbally, she had tried urinary anti-inflammatories (marsh mallow and corn silk), urinary antiseptics (cranberry juice and uva ursi), and urinary anodynes (hydrangea and gravel root). The herbs and the diet did little more than previous treatments with antibiotics, urethral dilation, and steroids.

Interstitial cystitis is a chronic inflammation of the bladder not caused by an infection. It primarily affects middle-aged women. The symptoms include frequent, painful urination; hematuria; and diminished urinary capacity. Although the cause of this condition is unknown, I believe it usually has an autoimmune component and/or one relating to food allergies. In this case, eliminating possible food triggers (including such common ones as wheat, dairy, citrus, beef, and soy) did not seem to result in any major improvements.

After reviewing what had previously been tried, I decided to focus my protocol on immune amphoterics to reduce hyperimmune response, herbs that drain heat in the bladder (anti-inflammatories), and urinary anodynes that I felt would be more appropriate. The following formula is a composite of several formulas used over 18 months: saw palmetto *(Serenoa repens)* 2 parts, ganoderma *(Ganoderma lucidum)* 2 parts, gardenia fruit *(Gardenia jasminoides)* 2 parts, eryngo *(Eryngium yuccafolium)* 1 part, and kava *(Piper methysticum)* 2 parts.

The first month, the patient thought she noted slight improvement, with a few days that were substantially better. Months two and three continued this trend except for a severe exacerbation between Christmas and New Year's. We believed this was primarily due to dramatic changes for the worse in her diet, alcohol consumption, and stress. By spring, the number of "good" days outnumbered those when the pain and irritation impinged on her quality of life. Throughout the summer and into the autumn, improvement was gradual but persistent. The last report I have had of this patient was that as long as she takes small maintenance doses of her herbs and doesn't radically change her diet, her condition isn't cured but is under control.

Case 4: Benign Prostatic Hyperplasia

The patient was a successful businessman, 61 years old, wealthy, a respected member of his church, and community, and a family man with three children and four grandchildren. On the surface everything was wonderful, but he had an embarrassing problem. Since his early 50s, he had started to experience signs of benign prostatic hyperplasia. At first, he ignored the more frequent urination, the need to get up at night to urinate, and the longer time it took to urinate. After a few years, the symptoms didn't go away; if anything, they became worse. His physician reassured him that the condition was common and could be treated, and prescribed Hytrin. Unfortunately, the medication not only didn't help his condition, it exacerbated his lifelong problem of feeling dizzy when he stood up quickly. Now he became dizzy when lying down, sitting up, and tying his shoes. This wasn't an acceptable solution. Next he received a prescription for Finasteride, and the dizziness improved but his prostate problems did not. Over the next few years, they became even worse. When his doctor mentioned the possibility of surgery, the patient decided it was time to look at other options. By the time I saw this apparently healthy, tall, and distinguished gentleman, he was getting up three to four times each night to urinate. Sometimes it took 10 to 15 minutes to urinate, and he never felt as if his bladder had completely emptied. Even worse was that his erections had become painful, and at the most inopportune times he would lose bladder control and dribble urine. He couldn't stand the thought that he might have to wear special undergarments to deal with the problem.

The protocol I designed for him included dietary supplements (zinc and omega-3 fatty acids), exercise (pelvic floor Kegel exercises), hydrotherapy (alternating hot and cold sitz baths), and an herbal formula. The herb formula consisted of 2 parts saw palmetto (S. repens), 1 part nettle root (Urtica dioica), 1 part aromatic collinsonia (Collinsonia canadensis), 1 part white sage (Salvia apiana), and 1 part agrimony (Agrimonia parviflora).

Within one month, there was definite improvement, less frequent urination, and a greater feeling of a fully emptied bladder. Month-by-month improvement was progressive, and by the six months, not only was the patient sleeping through most nights but his erections were no longer painful and his bladder control had returned. A visit to his physician was interesting when the doctor ascribed the improvements to a drug that the patient hadn't taken in over nine months.

These four cases are only a small sampling of many hundreds over the years that I have dealt with that were successful because they included saw palmetto as part of the protocol. That experience, plus the eclectic literature, has clearly proved to me that saw palmetto has a unique place in treating the reproductive problems of men and women, as well as immune deficiency, chronic lung problems, and — as we will show — a great deal more.

REPORTS FROM OTHER HERBALISTS

Wanting this book to be more than a recitation of historical uses, the current scientific data, and my personal experience, I invited some of the top herbalists and alternative practitioners in the United States and England to add their experience and comments.

Cascade Anderson–Geller, Herbalist

Cascade is the former chair of Botanical Medicine at the National College of Naturopathic Medicine in Portland, Oregon. She lectures throughout North and South America on the topic of herbal medicine and is the mother of two beautiful girls. She has used saw palmetto for urinary incontinence due to lack of tonicity in patients of all ages and both sexes. For loss of vaginal tonicity after multiple childbirths, she uses it with partridgeberry *(Mitchella repens)*. Cascade also uses *Serenoa* with herbs such as ginseng or gotu kola for weak, deficient, elderly people.

Ryan Drum, Ph.D., AHG

Dr. Drum is a biologist, a clinical herbalist, a popular lecturer, and probably America's premier wildcrafter. He presents some interesting food for thought with his experience.

"I initially used *Serenoa repens* tincture to loosen chronic respiratory mucus that was resistant to other herbal expectorants. The results were positive. The extract was made using 2 parts Korbel brandy to 1 part fresh ripe *Serenoa repens* whole berries in 2-quart jars. The crushed berries remained in the extract. Dosage was ½ ounce per day.

"For prostate, I use *Serenoa* tincture only when other herbs (*Equisetum*, *Solidago*, *Fucus*, *Epilobium*, Urtica root) and/or behavior modification fail, *and* when prostate swelling and discomfort are *not* caused by microbial infection. I believe *Serenoa* tincture helps expel watery mucopolypeptides from both the prostate gland and the respiratory tract.

"I am reluctant to use *Serenoa* extract because (a) It seems to reduce libido in my male patients with long-term (three-month) usage after an initial increase in libido at a dosage 5 milliliters per day; (b) it induces inappropriate disruption of testosterone metabolism when prostate distress originates from mechanical and/ or postural trauma; and (c) I wish to use it only when necessary.

"Anecdotal responses from prolonged *Serenoa* usage by men taking 5 milliliters a day include loss of chronic nonspecific anger, reduction in violent dream episodes, and a kinder attitude toward women, all of which tended to persist after *Serenoa* use was discontinued."

Author's note: Dr. Drum's experience is very interesting, but it is contradicted by eclectic usage and modern clinical research. This type of contrary data raises important questions and should be further studied by clinicians and researchers.

James Green, Herbalist

James is a clinical herbalist, medicine maker, author of *The Male Herbal,* and dean of the California School of Herbal Studies. He has specialized in male reproductive health issues. His experience with saw palmetto comes from a strong personal and clinical knowledge.

"Whenever I see a seemingly deficient, underdeveloped male or female individual who could benefit by a strengthened nervous system that will better support keener assimilation of nutrients, I feel very good recommending that they take the fruit of this plant as a food agent. I know it will nourish them in an essential and deeply satisfying way.

"I have experienced this personally with my own physical body, and I enjoyed the acquired inner substance that my being could begin to rely on. I certainly felt and looked more full-bodied and wholesome. I will share with you my work with a holistic urologist, a medical doctor who retired five years ago from 30 years of private practice.

"The doctor's patients (about 200 in number) were elderly men with prostate problems. The results with these gentlemen were 'much better than I would have ever expected, and I can relate this to my own personal experience as well. Many men who were getting up as much as four or five times at night to urinate are now getting up only once or twice. They state they are experiencing a quite noticeable improvement in the force and caliber of their urinary stream as well as a significant diminution in the time required to initiate the urinary body flow. In my experience so far, there doesn't seem to be any particular correlation between the size of the gland and the quality of the results. Also, many state that there is something inherently more satisfying about urination now.'

"I have been particularly gratified at the eagerness with which these older men (50s to 80s) have accepted taking an herb, and the determination they are showing about continuing."

Christopher Hedley, MNIMH

Christopher is a graduate of the School of Phytotherapy in England and maintains a clinical practice in London, England. He is the author of *Herbal Remedies,* a practical guide to making herbal remedies in the kitchen, and contributes articles to the *European Journal of Herbal Medicine.*

"I have used it for 'failure to thrive' in a child aged 3. This is, of course, the traditional use of the herb. He had very dry skin with a tendency to eczema and wheezing, with colds tending to go to his chest, which was diagnosed as asthma by his general practitioner. I disagreed with this diagnosis: asthma is grossly overdiagnosed in the UK, but that is another story. I gave him marsh mallow root tincture 3 parts and saw palmetto tincture 1 part, with instructions to give 5 milliliters (100 drops) two times per day. This was continued, with other herbs added according to his symptoms, for 18 months and was spectacularly successful."

Christopher Hobbs, L.Ac., AHG

Christopher Hobbs is a fourth-generation herbalist and botanist with over 20 years of experience with herbs. He is a prolific author, lectures throughout the world, and maintains a busy practice in Santa Cruz, California.

"Carol was a 40-year-old woman who came into my office six months ago complaining of burning with urination, increased urge to urinate, and a feeling of pressure over her lower abdominal area. She told me she had had problems with recurring bladder infections for over five years. As a practitioner of traditional Chinese medicine and as a Western herbalist, I wanted to make a diagnosis based on her present condition and not just treat her symptoms. To help with the diagnosis I looked at her tongue, felt her pulse, reviewed Carol's diet, and felt her lower abdominal area for tension and tenderness. Carol's tongue had a thick greasy yellow coating toward the back, showing accumulation of dampness and excessive heat in her bowels and other lower abdominal organs. Her pulse was full and slightly fast. I detected no sign of weakness, and she confirmed that she was rarely fatigued. Her lower abdomen was tense and painful.

"Based on these signs, I gave her an herbal formula to clear the heat and dampness, and asked her if she was willing to cut way back on her intake of simple sugars, sticking only to fresh fruit in season. She also agreed to cut her coffee and caffeine intake to a bare minimum. Sugar and stimulants activate the body's metabolism and often aggravate the accumulation of dampness and heat in the body.

"I gave Carol a formula with burdock root, yellow dock root, dandelion root, and about 20% *Cascara sagrada* to clear the dampness and heat. Carol took the formula for two weeks, stuck to her diet, then returned to the clinic. Her tongue still had a yellow coat, but the coating was much thinner, and her general tongue appearance looked better. Most of her bladder symptoms had also disappeared. At this stage I gave Carol saw palmetto capsules, each containing 320 milligrams of standardized hexane-free extract. I asked her to take one capsule in the morning and one in the evening. I have had good luck with this high dose, but 160 milligrams once or twice a day works for some patients.

"Carol came back after 1 month and reported very good success with the diet and herbal program. She had no further burning or other symptoms of bladder infection. Two months later she came in again and was very impressed with the positive results she had had with the saw palmetto. During the previous five years she had constantly had a bladder infection, but not after starting with saw palmetto.

"I have excellent results with saw palmetto for relieving nighttime urination and pain with benign prostatic hyperplasia in men. I often give a double dose for best results for the first few months, then cut to a normal dose. My clinical experience with other women shows that saw palmetto is not just a men's herb. I find saw palmetto to be excellent for strengthening the genitourinary tract and reducing irritation and inflammation in both men and women."

Tieraona Low Dog, M.D., AHG

Dr. Low Dog is a clinical herbalist, a medical doctor, an exceptionally compelling lecturer, and dean of the Foundations of Herbal Medicine Program in Albuquerque, New Mexico.

"I have had some female patients with subjective improvement with their hirsutism brought about by polycystic ovary disease. This may be due in part to the fact that 5-alpha-reductase is elevated in women with that condition. I have also had far more success with *Serenoa* than with Vitex in the treatment of acne. Women with estrogen excess and acne during the luteal phase of the menstrual cycle do particularly well with this herb. While the standardized extract seems to work better, I have still had results with a 1:1 fluid extract."

Amanda McQuade Crawford, B.A., MNIMH, AHG

Amanda was trained at the School of Phytotherapy in England. She is an educator, practitioner, and lecturer, and she speaks throughout the United States, England, Australia, and New Zealand. Amanda also is the author of *Herbal Remedies for Women* and *The Herbal Menopause Book*.

"When I began in practice, a young woman came as a patient with a breast lesion that had first been diagnosed as Paget's disease but then was reclassified as benign without any clear diagnosis. After seeing several physicians over several months, and before her appointment with me, the woman sought advice from a psychic, who recommended she take saw palmetto. When I heard this, I (who "knew all about" *Serenoa repens*) rolled my eyes to heaven for mercy but maintained my composure with my patient. She had already been taking 560-milligram capsules three times a day for three weeks. I asked her to put them aside during the course of our herbal treatment. I went straight home to my library, looked up *Serenoa*, and found nineteenth-century literature suggesting its use for female breast complaints, especially lesions, that resisted both certain diagnosis and treatment by other means. I asked all psychics for pardon on the etheric plane, and the patient improved after resuming the use of saw palmetto."

Michelle Pouliot, N.D.

Michelle graduated from Bastyr College in 1991 and from International Foundation of Homeopathy in 1993. She has a B.S. in biochemistry and is a naturopathic physician in Torrington, Connecticut, with a busy clinical practice. She uses herbal medicine, homeopathy, nutrition, and physiotherapy. She has used the standardized extract of saw palmetto successfully for the treatment of deep cystic acne in women in their 20s and 30s. She has also found it useful for polycystic ovary syndrome.

"Herbal" Ed Smith, Herbalist AHG

Herbal Ed is the founder of one of the premier herbal manufacturers in the United States, Herb Pharm. Ed is a popular lecturer, has taught extensively at the naturopathic colleges in Washington State and Oregon, and travels throughout the world researching herbal medicine.

"A woman, who was a neighbor, had a champion show dog with severe benign prostatic hyperplasia. Her veterinarian suggested a prostatectomy for this chronic condition. This was unacceptable, as the dog's owner received substantial income from the dog's stud fee. The dog was given saw palmetto and vitamin E, which reduced the symptoms and the need for surgery. Over the next few years the dog sired many more puppies."

Terry Willard, Ph.D., AHG

Dr. Willard is a clinical herbalist who has practiced since 1975. He is the author of eight books on herbal medicine and a CD-ROM, *The Interactive Herbal.* He is a popular lecturer, the president of the Canadian Association of Herbal Practitioners, and the president of Wild Rose College of Natural Healing in Calgary, Alberta. Dr. Willard finds that saw palmetto seems to be more effective in the spring and summer than in the autumn or winter months. He theorizes that this is because the liver meridian, which is more active in the spring, passes through the prostate, increasing circulation of blood and Qi. Dr. Willard also has noticed that saw palmetto helps with what he calls "grumpy old man syndrome." He feels that the increased androgens and hormonal shifts of middle age, sometimes designated male menopause, create increased aggression and irritability. In his clinic, not only have men reported a more relaxed feeling — so have their loved ones!

Donald Yance, AHG, C.N.

Donald Yance is a well-respected clinical herbalist who specializes in treating patients with chronic degenerative diseases. He is the author of *Herbal Medicine, Healing and Cancer* and he maintains two very busy practices and healing centers in Oregon and Connecticut. Donald is well versed in the eclectic traditions and in modern scientific research. He has effectively used saw palmetto for pattern balding in both men and women, and he feels it is especially effective for infertility in women who have elevated androgens with hirsutism (excess hair on the face).

From these practitioners' accounts it becomes obvious that among highly skilled clinicians, saw palmetto is used in a much wider scope than is reported in the popular literature. Both traditional uses and experimental new uses continue to enlarge the current narrow vision that has, for many years, limited saw palmetto's usefulness.

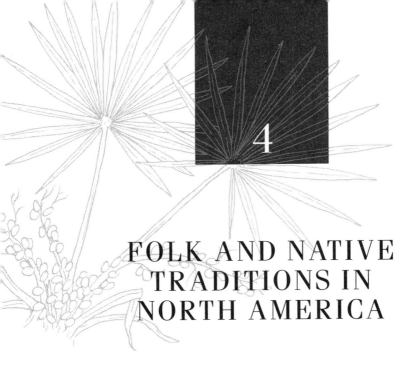

FOLK AND NATIVE
TRADITIONS IN
NORTH AMERICA

Native people of North America, as well as European settlers here, found many uses for saw palmetto to benefit their way of life. The leaves of this small palm tree were used extensively for thatch to create long-lasting waterproof roofs and shelters. It appears that the strong fiber-bearing leaves were so valued by native people that they traded them throughout the country; archeologists have found the remnants of various palm species far beyond their natural range.

PRACTICAL USES

The Winnebago used palm leaves to produce cordage for bags. The Iroquois are known to have used palm leaf fiber for burden straps, and the Cherokee used the leaves to create durable baskets. The Mikasuki Seminoles, who live in Florida where this palm grows, call it *sheope taale*. They use the leaves to make medicine baskets, rope, dance fans, rattles, fire fans, fish nets, and the famous Seminole dolls, as well as for tinder. Southern craftpersons have recently used them to make fans, brooms, hats, baskets, chair seats, and mattress fillings. For a time in the late 1800s, the leaves were made into a strong, tear-resistant paper that yielded writing paper or stationery, but it was considered to be of a poor quality.

The stems and root fibers of this palm have been used as a source of the chemical tannin, which is used in tanning animal hides, as a cork substitute, and as a fiber for strengthening wallboard during World War II.

European settlers used the tangled roots of saw palmetto as scrub brushes, and the roots were burned to create potash salts as a source of alkali. The seeds yield a fixed oil (a nonvolatile vegetable oil), which burns cleanly with a blue flame that gives off a peculiar coffee-like odor. A wax extracted from the leaves was investigated as a source of industrial vegetable wax, but it was found to be less useful than already available sources.

In Florida, the flowers of saw palmetto provide a major source of good-quality seasonal nectar for honeybees, and they attract butterflies as well.

The fruits (drupes) are eagerly eaten by wild animals (bear, deer, raccoon, possums, fish, and waterbirds), and early settlers used them to feed hogs, goats, and poultry. In fact, interest in using the berries for medicine was sparked by people noticing how fat and healthy the animals who fed on saw palmetto became. According to a recent article by Bennett and Hicklin in the journal *Economic Botany*, saw palmetto provides food or cover for more then 100 birds, 27 mammals, 25 amphibians, and 61 reptile species.

In the late nineteenth century, a carbonated beverage called Metto was made with the berries. This soft drink was sold at roadside stands in Miami. If you have ever tasted the berries, it doesn't require much imagination to understand why this product inevitably failed. Several texts mention the use of saw palmetto berries in "aromatizing" cognac. The resulting product would, I am sure, be an acquired taste.

Berries as Food

There is ample evidence of indigenous use of the berries for food. To the Western taste the berries are strongly disagreeable, first coming across as sweet, then having a strong acrid and pungent secondary taste. Early colonists experienced the unique taste of saw palmetto berries when they were shipwrecked on the Florida coast.

There is no doubt that the aborigines of the Florida peninsula depended largely on the berries of the saw palmetto for their food. A very old book, narrated by Jonathan Dickinson and published in 1796, describes the adventures of a shipload of Quakers who were shipwrecked on the coast of Florida at its extreme southern point in August 1696. They were captured by the Indians, who were believed to be cannibals. After terrible sufferings on the part of the men and women, they arrived at St. Augustine. Dickinson narrates that on their arrival they were taken to the wigwam of the "casseky," or chief, who "seated himself in his cabin, cross-legged, having a basket of palmetto berries brought him, which he ate very greedily." These Quakers, nearly starved to death while they were with the Indians. The only food given them were fish and berries. Their first trial of the berries was not favorable. "We tasted them, but not one among us could suffer them to stay in our mouths, for we could compare the taste of them to nothing else but *rotten cheese steeped in tobacco juice.*"

Seeds and Bud

African Americans of the West Indies traditionally were said to grind the hard white seeds into a flour that was baked into a crude bread or porridge. The terminal bud can be eaten as a vegetable and is considered superior to the traditional hearts of palm *(Sabal palmetto).* Lee Peterson, in his classic *Field Guide to Edible Wild Plants,* says that the palm heart is "firm textured, yet tender and makes an excellent salad or cooked vegetable." Readers should be aware that harvesting this part of the plant will kill it. Fortunately with the tremendous abundance of saw palmetto (almost weed status), judicious harvesting is unlikely to damage the plant's population.

EARLY INDIGENOUS USES AS MEDICINE

I believe it is very likely that the original indigenous peoples of Florida, the Timucua, the Tequesta, the Calusa, and the Apalache, used saw palmetto berries for medicine, but there is almost no written record of such usage. Because of early contacts with Spanish and English explorers, this indigenous culture and its accumulated wisdom were destroyed by disease, enslavement, and genocide. The people who had knowledge of local plant uses were long gone by the time the dominant culture became interested in recording the uses of native plants.

Arnold Krochmal, Ph.D., in his book *Medicinal Plants of the United States,* briefly mentions Gulf Coast Indians who made an infusion of the leaves and roots for dysentery and for relieving stomach pain. From the inner trunk bark, they also made poultices for insect and snake bites and skin ulcers. The Houma of Louisiana used a decoction of the root for sore eyes, high blood pressure, and kidney problems. The fruits of closely related species of palms have been used as medicine throughout the Caribbean and the Yucatan in Mexico. Sabal japa fruit bears a close resemblance to the fruit of saw palmetto; an extract of that fruit is used as a sedative and digestive stimulant. It was also used for respiratory problems and for weakness of the reproductive system.

ORIGINS OF WESTERN MEDICAL USE

While saw palmetto may have been used in folk medicine, not until the 1870s was it introduced into Western medical practice. A Dr. J. B. Reed of Savannah, Georgia, first wrote about the medicinal uses of *Serenoa* in 1877 in an article published in *The Medical Brief.* Dr.

Reed claimed that saw palmetto berries improved digestion, nutrition, and strength and relieved irritation of the mucous membranes, especially those of the nose and bronchial passages. He mentioned successful treatment of bronchial catarrh, ozena, chronic coughs, and bronchitis. He stated:

Considering the great and diversified power of the saw palmetto as a therapeutic agent, it seems strange that it should have so long escaped the notice of the medical profession. Several years ago, while on a hunting expedition in the wilds of Florida, my attention was called to the great fattening properties of the berries, and the peculiar quality of the fat of animals that feed on them. Most animals in the palmetto regions are very fond of the fruit. During the summer months in these parts, the supply of fruit is scarce for such animals as bears, raccoons, opossums and hogs, and they have to work hard to eke out a living from roots and such animal foods as they can find upon the sea coast such as turtle eggs, dead fish, etc. and they consequently become very thin. As soon, however, as the palmetto berries begin to ripen they improve rapidly, and in a few weeks have acquired an enormous quantity of fat, so as to become so unwieldy that they are an easy prey to the hunter. This fat, like that of mast-eating animals, consists principally of olein, and will not make lard. The berries, when dropped into water, are seized and eaten with avidity by the fishes. Even the natives frequently acquire a taste for the berries, and eat them freely. It is the only thing, it is claimed, that will fatten a piny woods razor-back hog.

An eclectic physician, Dr. I. J. M. Goss of Marietta, Georgia, next mentioned the use of these oily berries. He made claims supporting Dr. Reed's experience. Further testimony to the effects of *Serenoa* were published by a pharmacist, J. M. Dixon, in the *Pacific Record of Medicine and Surgery* (circa 1880). Another physician, Dr. F. A. Evans, reported in *The Medical Brief* (circa 1885) that he had found that 15 minims (approximately 15 drops) of the fluid extract of saw palmetto would stop the paroxysm of migraine.

Saw palmetto is a sedative, nutrient and diuretic. It improves digestion, induces sleep, increases flesh and weight and strength. It relieves irritation of the mucous membrane of the throat, nose and larynx, and controls and cures purulent discharges from the mucous membrane. The fluid extract of this valuable berry, as a nutrient tonic, is far in advance of the compound hypophosphites, but has a special action on the glands of the reproductive organs, as the mammae, ovaries, prostate, testes, etc. Its action is that of a great vitalizer, tending to increase their activity, to promote their secreting faculty, and adding greatly to their size.

It is specially indicated in all cases of wasting of the testes, which is often present in sexual impotency. In atrophy of the prostate, this drug operates in a most remarkable manner in overcoming the withered, blighted state of the gland; also in uterine atrophy, dependent upon ovarian blight, its action is unexcelled. In gynecological practice it is much used to promote the growth of the mammae, but it is on the prostate gland that this remedy exercises its best effects.

A physician, Stephen F. Dupore, M.D., of Savannah, Georgia, was quoted in an 1880 issue of the *Therapeutic Gazette:*

Perhaps no remedy yet brought forward has met with more positive good results in diseases affecting the throat, bronchial tubes and lungs. Whooping cough in the first stage has been cut off. In another case, that of hemorrhage of the lungs, it checked it at once. In aphonia, this remedy restores the voice in a few hours.

Many physicians also believed that this herb could be used to treat and restore vitality for patients suffering from tuberculosis.

Widespread Acceptance by 1890s

By the late 1880s and early 1890s, the use of saw palmetto in eclectic, homeopathic, and allopathic medicine had become widespread. The berries were listed in the official medical literature starting in the 1890s; they were first listed in the 17th edition of the *U.S. Dispensatory* in 1894 and continued to be listed until the 25th edition in 1955. The berries were official in the *U.S. Pharmacopoeia* from 1906 to 1916 and then in the *National Formulary* from 1926 to 1950.

Saw palmetto also gained recognition in the British literature. In 1916, it was listed in the 19th edition of *Squire's Companion to the British Pharmacopoeia* as an admixture of sandlewood. It was given a substantial clinical monograph in the *British Pharmaceutical Codex* of 1923 and more recently in the *British Herbal Pharmacopoeia,* published in 1979.

ECLECTIC TRADITION

The eclectics were a popular sectarian medical group that existed from the 1830s through the 1940s. They were founded by Dr. Wooster Beach, M.D., as an alternative to the dangerous heroic medical practices of the early nineteenth century (bleeding and the use of calomel, mercury, arsenic, and opium). The eclectic physicians primarily used herbal remedies to treat disease, and they focused on studying and using the "American Vegetable Materia Medica." As mentioned previously, a Southern eclectic, Dr. I. J. M. Goss, first introduced the use of *Serenoa* to his eclectic brethren. Their experience with this herb broadened its scope of usage. Felter and Lloyd, in the 18th edition of *King's Dispensatory,* credited the berries with being a "superior" nutritive tonic, stimulating the appetite and improving digestion and assimilation. They also spoke highly of its use for irritation of the mucous membranes, such as that caused by irritative cough, chronic bronchial cough, pertussis (whooping cough), acute and chronic laryngitis, acute catarrh, and asthma.

For genitourinary tract conditions, the authors claimed that many experienced practitioners had found this herb effective for irritation associated with gonorrhea, orchitis, epididymitis, and ovarian pain. Although they did not use the term, they described saw palmetto as a reproductive amphoteric (an amphoteric is a substance that normalizes function, via its nutritive qualities). While it was used for prostatic enlargement, it was also recommended for atrophied breasts, testes, and ovaries.

Herbert T. Webster, M.D., a prominent eclectic physician from California, mentioned the following clinical insight for saw palmetto in his superb text *Dynamical Therapeutics*. He used the tincture of the semifresh berries for relaxation of the urinary organs with exhaustion of the nervous system, frequent urination, and vesical irritation with prostatic hypertrophy. In his text, he related a case history in which he used *Serenoa* for female reproductive problems. He successfully used the berries for inflammation of the fallopian tubes with concurrent ovarian pain. Further symptoms included a dragging sensation in the pelvis and abdominal tenderness with a mucopurulent discharge.

Other prominent eclectic physicians mentioned additional therapeutic uses. J. W. Fyfe, M.D., in *Specific Diagnosis and Specific Medication*, advocated this herb for irritation of the nose, throat, pharynx, and larynx. He found that inhalation of the vapor was useful for sinus congestion, postnasal drip, and bronchial catarrh. He also suggested that the berries be used as a general bladder tonic to strengthen function and tonicity.

In the *Medical Gleaner* (1897), an eclectic medical journal that focused on materia medica and therapeutics, Dr. J. D. Hatton highly commended the use of saw palmetto for the symptoms of chronic gonorrhea. He stated that this herb was more than satisfactory at relieving the discharge and removing irritation, usually in as little as three or four days.

Eli G. Jones, one of the most "eclectic" of physicians (he was trained as an eclectic, homeopath, physiomedicalist, and allopathic physician), felt that saw palmetto was very useful for deficient impotence (sexual neurasthenia), loss of libido, infertility due to overwork (stress), exhaustion, and excessive childbearing. His symptom picture for prostate problems was succinct and accurate: chronic prostatitis or enlargement of the gland with throbbing, aching, dull pain, and difficult, often painful urination.

In the scarce *Journal of the North American Eclectic Materia Medica Association,* mention was made of a similarity between the tissue of the "prostate and the tonsils." Because of this perceived similarity, the herb was recommended as a useful remedy for chronic inflammation of the tonsils, croup, snoring, and chronic sore throat.

HOMEOPATHIC PRACTICES

Another form of medical practice that flourished during the late nineteenth century, and continues today, is homeopathy. Homeopathy (*Homeo:* similar, *pathos:* suffering) was created in 1796 by a physician, Samual Hahneman, in Germany. It flourished throughout Europe and was introduced in the United States in 1825 by Hans Burch Gram, M.D., a Danish physician. Saw palmetto was first introduced to the homeopathic profession by the work of two women. The first "proving" (study) of *Serenoa* was made by a lay homeopath, Annie Roash. Her provings showed a strong action of saw palmetto on the breasts, head, and ovaries. The second study was made by Dr. Freda Langton of Omaha, Nebraska, who found strong indications for using the remedy for conditions of the mind, bladder, ovaries, and uterus.

In 1898, Edwin M. Hale, M.D., collected all the known information on this herb in his book *Saw Palmetto, Its History, Botany, Chemistry, Pharmacology, Provings, Clinical Experience and Therapeutic Applications.* Hale mentioned multiple preparations made with *Serenoa.* He used a simple fresh tincture, as well as a fluid extract made from the fresh "green" berries (which he felt was four times stronger than the tincture). An oil was made by allowing the expressed juice to stand for a few days, after which the juice was mixed with cane sugar to make a saccharated oil. The saccharated oil was primarily used in lozenges for irritative throat problems. Hale also made a preparation called *aqua olei sabal* by combining the oil with magnesium carbonate and water. This product was used as a spray for the sinuses, tonsils, and throat.

Homeopathic Indications

The homeopathic indications for saw palmetto to some degree mirror those of the eclectics but included a few widely divergent uses as well. Dr. Boericke, in the ninth edition of his classic text *Pocket Manual of Homeopathic Materia Medica,* published in 1927, listed the following symptom pictures, or indications, for the medicine *Serenoa.*

Symptoms affecting the mind: emotional disturbance and irritability caused by a direct influence from the reproductive function, i.e., premenstrual syndrome depression, dysmenorrhea with irritability, menopausal cloudy thinking, headache from mental strain or menses.

Symptoms affecting the head, ears, and nose: headache with vertigo, pain in the temples and the top of the head, inflammation of the middle ear, sneezing, constant postnasal drip with coughing and gagging.

Symptoms affecting the mouth, throat, and bronchials: pungent burning sensation in the mouth and throat, hoarseness, pharyngeal cough, croupy cough, chronic bronchitis with depletion and poor digestion.

Symptoms affecting the urinary organs: poor bladder control, irritation caused by gonorrhea, burning urination, dysuria, constantly sensation of overfull bladder.

Symptoms affecting the male reproductive organs: testicular atrophy, feelings of fullness in the bladder and pressure to urinate with some tenderness and soreness over bladder, enlarged prostate gland with cutting pains on urinating or inability to urination with heat and fullness, loss of libido, backache after ejaculation.

Symptoms affecting the female reproductive organs: vesicle irritation; tender enlarged ovaries; stooping walk caused by the tenderness; extreme fatigue, usually from overindulgence; atrophy of the breasts; stinging pain in the breasts during nursing.

Generalities: feebleness with weakness, anorexia, cachexia, and emaciation.

External uses of serenoa oil: as an application for psoriasis, swollen joints, enlarged lymph nodes, and alopeica.

According to Dr. John H. Clarke, in his *Dictionary of Materia Medica,* homeopathic Silica and Pulsatilla are contraindicated in a patient taking saw palmetto, as they antidote the remedy. An early homeopathic physician, Elias C. Price, M.D., recorded several unusual case histories in which *Serenoa* was used. One patient was a very nervous woman with chronic inflammation of the bladder. She had frequent and painful urination, 10 to 20 times per night and every 15 to 30 minutes during the day. A rectal examination revealed a hard fleshy tumor the size of half a hen's egg on the posterior of the uterus. She was given *Sabal (Serenoa)* fluid extract, five drops, three times per day. In two months the tumor was reduced in size by half, and after another three months the tumor and the urinary problem were entirely resolved. In other cases, Dr. Price successfully used *Sabal* for pelvic cellulitis; peritonitis; puerperal fever; inflammation of the uterus, fallopian tubes, and ovaries; and even appendicitis.

PHYSIOMEDICAL USES

The physiomedicalists were yet another sectarian medical group in the United States that was founded by Alva Curtis, M.D., in 1839. Descended from the Thomsonians of the early nineteenth century, they eschewed the use of any toxic remedies. Even more than the eclectics, physiomedical practitioners relied almost exclusively on herbs as therapeutic agents. Saw palmetto was first noted in their literature at the rather late date of 1896.

Dr. William Cook, in his book *A Compend of the Newer Materia Medica,* recounted the accepted uses of *Serenoa:* "It influences the sensory and sympathetic nerve peripheries, the mucous membranes and reproductive organs of both sexes." T. J. Lyle, M.D., in his textbook *Physio-Medical Therapeutics, Materia Medica and Pharmacy,* also reinforced the prevailing uses of *Serenoa.* He noted an interesting formula for a saw palmetto compound that he recommended as an excellent tonic diuretic; the ingredients were *Serenoa,* parsley, cola nut, sandalwood, and essential oils.

POPULAR AND FOLK TRADITIONS

In popular and folk medicine, saw palmetto has been used widely since the 1880s. Numerous patent medicines were available around the turn of the century. Palmetto wine, a combination of orange juice and *Serenoa,* was sold and promoted in Florida for sexual neurasthenia. The OD Chemical Company produced Sanmetto, a combination of saw palmetto and sandalwood, in a flavored base. It was recommended for benign prostatic hypertropy, urethral inflammation, irritable bladder, and ovarian pain, and it continued to be sold until the 1930s.

Early Twentieth Century Formulas

Numerous ethical drug companies also had saw palmetto-based formulas for similar problems. The Tilden Company, which had started producing herbal medicines in New Lebanon, New York, in 1824, listed three saw palmetto formulas in its 1937 catalog, including a saw palmetto compound that contained *Serenoa,* sandalwood, kola nut, and celery seed.

John Wyeth and Brother of Philadelphia, in a 1901 catalog, listed a saw palmetto compound that also contained kola nut, parsley seed, and coca leaves. They recommend it for urinary complaints, prostatic irritation, and catarrhal conditions, and as an aphrodisiac. Major pharmaceutical companies, including Lilly, Squibb, and Merck, all produced products from this aromatic berry.

Popular Herbals

Popular herbals throughout the twentieth century have generally echoed the earlier uses of this herb. Jethro Kloss, in his classic book *Back to Eden,* says the berries are useful for respiratory problems and reproductive diseases, and he mentions an unusual use as a remedy for diabetes and Bright's disease. Maude Grieve, in her impressive and influential text *A Modern Herbal,* states that saw palmetto acts on the urinary and respiratory tissue but is milder and less stimulant than cubeb or copaiba or even oil of sandalwood. Alma Hutchens, in her peculiar but popular *Indian Herbology of North America,* boldly states that saw palmetto is one of the "most beneficial agents of the Materia Medica." The uses in her book closely follow the suggestions found in Jethro Kloss's earlier book.

USING SAW PALMETTO FOR PROSTATE HEALTH
Approaches and Formulas

Many clinical studies of saw palmetto have been done throughout the world. Most if not all of them have used the standardized 85 to 95 percent fatty acid extract. This type of product is preferred for studies, as it is consistent in activity and quality, thus reducing a possible variable that could invalidate test results. Some authors and lecturers claim that only this form of *Serenoa* is effective. This is patently false! No studies of the standardized extract comparing it with tincture, capsule or tea have ever been done. Thus, there is no proof of its greater activity. In fact, it is because of the long and continued use of nonstandardized teas, tinctures, and capsules containing saw palmetto that researchers became interested in studying this herb for prostate problems.

STANDARDIZED HERBAL PRODUCTS

Be aware that the concerted push for standardization in the herbal marketplace has more to do with the manufacturers' desire to be accepted by the orthodox medical community and by the consumer, and a lack of true understanding about herbal medicine, than it does with quality. Some "standardized" products are standardized to mediocrity rather than to exceptional quality. There are other problems with some standardized extracts, including solvent residues (hexane) and concentration of chemical pollutants (pesticides, herbicides, fungicides) found on the commercial-grade herbs used in making these products. There is a place in herbal medicine for highly concentrated preparations (phytopharmaceuticals), but these products should not be confused with traditional herbal medicines. There is a trade-off: certain activities may be enhanced, but other qualities may be greatly reduced or lost entirely. Some phytopharmaceuticals have a more "drug-like" activity, and this may increase the possibility of drug/herb interactions or adverse reactions.

An example of this problem is provided by the herbal medicine turmeric. It has been used in India for thousands of years as a spice, in curry, and as a powerful medicine. In recent years, researchers had isolated one ingredient in turmeric, curcumin (ker-coo-min), and believed that it was the active ingredient. Studies on standardized 90 percent curcumin extracts have shown active anti-inflammatory, antihepatotoxin, antioxidant, and antimutagenic activity. The whole root and whole root extract have since been found to have other active constituents in addition to curcumin, including essential oils and water-based compounds. These substances may add significant activity to the herb, but they are mostly or totally missing in the curcumin product. The other major difference is that the turmeric extracts have protective effect on the gastric mucosa, while high doses of curcumin have been linked to increased gastric irritation and ulceration.

In the case of saw palmetto, the standardized extract may have a greater activity in conditions such as benign prostatic hyperplasia/hypertrophy (BPH), cystic acne, male pattern baldness, and female hirsutism. At the same time, this type of product has little or no activity as an immune potentiator, adaptogen, lung tonic, or reproductive amphoteric.

RELIEVING SYMPTOMS OF BENIGN PROSTATIC HYPERPLASIA

Modern clinical use of saw palmetto has mainly focused on its ability to relieve the symptoms associated with BPH. This condition, also known as prostatism or adenoma of the prostate, is a common nonmalignant enlargement of the prostate that occurs in middle-aged men. Most men aged 45 or older have some enlargement of this gland, which surrounds the neck of the bladder and the urethra. In addition to the swelling of the tissue, the texture of the gland change. Small nodules can develop, changing the shape and size of this normally chestnut-sized gland, reducing flexibility and bladder control.

Symptoms and Causes of Benign Prostatic Hyperplasia

The symptoms usually begin in men during their late 50s or early 60s, and the condition tends to be progressive. Symptoms can include urinary frequency, difficulty urinating, dribbling of urine, reduction of the urinary stream, incomplete emptying of the bladder, and occasionally urinary retention. While the condition is not dangerous, it can have a strong impact on quality of life. Nighttime urinary frequency can seriously disrupt sleep, and incomplete emptying of the bladder can increase the likelihood of urinary tract infections. The later stages of BPH (Vahlensieck's stages 3 and 4 — see page 56) are more serious, as complete blockage of urine can occur, with back-pressure of urine causing kidney damage and uremia.

Current medical theory suggests that the primary cause of prostatic swelling is an increased production of the potent androgen dihydrotestosterone (DHT). While testosterone levels drop with increased age, follicle-stimulating hormone (FSH), luteinizing hormone (LH), prolactin, and estradiol steadily increase. The elevated levels of estrogens decrease metabolism of DHT, and increased prolactin also raises the levels of DHT in the prostate.

The belief that DHT is a major culprit in BPH is supported by the fact that men with deficiencies of DHT do not have prostatic enlargement. The increased levels of estrogens (estradiol), compared with testosterone in aging men, suggest that estrogen (including environmental estrogens from pesticides, plastics, chlorine, etc.) may also have a role to play in BPH. The combination of all of these factors — age-related physiologic changes, the Western diet, and environmental pollutants (cadmium, exogenous estrogens) — triggers the overstimulation and growth of prostatic tissue and the troublesome symptoms associated with prostate problems. Certain medications and foods, including alcohol, coffee, amphetamines, and antihistamines, may exacerbate this condition.

VAHLENSIECK'S CLASSIFICATION OF BENIGN PROSTATIC HYPERPLASIA (BPH)

Pharmacological treatment (drugs or herbs) is most effective for stage 1 and stage 2 symptoms and may also have some benefit for stage 3 symptoms. Stage 3 and stage 4 symptoms are most appropriately treated by surgical intervention.

STAGE 1 SYMPTOMS	STAGE 2 SYMPTOMS	STAGE 3 SYMPTOMS	STAGE 4 SYMPTOMS
Normal micturition	Periodic disturbances of micturition	Permanent disturbances of micturition	Permanent disturbances of micturition
Moderate hyperplasia	Moderate hyperplasia	Hyperplasia	Hyperplasia
Urine flow over 15 milliliters per second	Urine flow between 10 and 15 milliliters per second	Urine flow under 10 milliliters per second	Urine flow under 10 milliliters per second
No residual urine	Residual urine under 50 milliliters	Residual urine over 50 milliliters	Residual urine over 50 milliliters
No "trabecula" bladder	No, or only initial evidences of, "trabecula" bladder	"Trabecula" bladder	Dilated bladder
			Residual urine in the upper urinary tract

From *Fitoterapia* 68(3), 1997

CLINICAL STUDIES OF THE EFFECTIVENESS OF SERENOA EXTRACT

The exact mechanism of action exerted by saw palmetto on prostatic tissue is unclear. Many early in-vitro studies claimed that its effects were due in part to its ability to inhibit an enzyme, 5-alpha-reductase, which is responsible for converting testosterone into DHT. Later studies, however, showed that Serenoa has only a weak inhibitory action on this enzyme. In fact, in-vitro studies comparing *Serenoa* extract's ability to inhibit 5-alpha-reductase to finasteride showed it to be 5,600 times weaker.

A study by W. Breu and M. Hagenlocher, published in the German journal *Arzneim-Forsch Drug Research* in 1992, used a supercritical carbon dioxide extract of saw palmetto. The researchers were exploring the mechanism of action of this herb for benign prostatic hyperplasia. Most research has studied and confirmed the ability of *Serenoa* to inhibit 5-alpha-reductase and reduce the formation of DHT. The researchers in this experiment found another mechanism of action for saw palmetto: inhibition of the biosynthesis of inflammatory arachadonic acid metabolites, specifically the cyclooxygenase and 5-lipoxgenase pathways.

According to Italian researchers Professors Bombardelli and Morazzoni, as published in *Fitoterapia* in 1997, possible mechanisms of action for *Serenoa* include the following:

1. Inhibition 5-alpha-reductase, thereby
   a. inhibiting conversion of testosterone to DHT;
   b. this in turn reduces the level of DHT in the bloodstream.
2. Inhibition of aromatase, which stimulates the conversion of testosterone to estradiol;
   a. this lowers the levels of DHT in the prostate.
3. Decrease in the activity of estrogen receptors in the prostate.
4. Inhibition of phospholipase A2,
   a. which inhibits free arachadonic acid,
   b. which reduces inflammation.

5. Inhibition of 5-lipoxygenase enzymes,
   a. which inhibits arachadonic acid,
   b. which reduces inflammation.
6. Inhibition of cyclooxygenase pathways,
   a. which inhibits arachadonic acid,
   b. which reduces inflammation.
7. Spasmolytic activity,
   a. which increases prostate muscle tone and reduces atonic tissue.
8. Inhibition of fibroblastic growth factor (FGF) and epithelium growth factor (EGF),
   a. which would reduce prostate growth and inflammation.
9. Inhibition of the prostate's uptake of the hormone prolactin,
   a. which may inhibit prolactin-induced prostate growth.

Beyond the effects noted above, studies show that the extract of *Serenoa* appears to lack any direct estrogenic activity, effect on the pituitary, or progestational effects.

Evidence of Effectiveness

Following are summaries of five significant studies that clearly show the activity and effectiveness of *Serenoa* extract for BPH.

1. Braeckman et al. "The Extract of *Serenoa repens* in the Treatment of Benign Prostatic Hyperplasia." In this three-month multicenter open study, 505 patients took 160 milligrams twice a day of *Serenoa* extract. The efficiency of the treatment was measured using the International Prostate Symptom Score, the Quality of Life Score, urinary flow rates, residual urine volume, and prostate size. After 45 days of treatment, there was significant improvement. After 90 days of this therapy, 88 percent of patients and physicians considered saw palmetto to be effective. In addition, the serum prostate specific antigen (PSA) concentration was not modified by the herb, thus limiting the risk of masking the possible development of prostate cancer during treatment. The incidence of side effects was low (5 percent), and all side effects were minor.

2. Vahlensieck et al. "Benign Prostatic Hyperplasia: Treatment with Sabal Fruit Extract." This large study conducted on 1,334 patients with BPH lasted twelve weeks. While under treatment, the volume of residual urine decreased on average by 37 percent and nocturea by 54 percent. The percentage of patients with dysuric pain was reduced from 75 percent to 37 percent. More than 80 percent of the patients rated the treatment good to excellent and 95 percent of them tolerated saw palmetto well.

3. Champault et al. "Medical treatment of Prostatic Adenoma." One hundred and ten patients with a prostatic adenoma that needed medical treatment but did not require surgery were treated in a controlled study. The month-long test was judged on objective (nocturnal pollakiuria, urinary output, residual urine) and subjective criteria (dysuria, patients' opinions). *Serenoa* showed significantly greater effectiveness than placebo and was perfectly tolerated. Supplementary studies in 47 patients with a mean follow-up of 14.6 months showed continued effectiveness and lack of side effects.

4. Duvia et al. "Advances in the Phytotherapy of Prostatic Hypertrophy." The effectiveness and tolerability of saw palmetto extract was compared with pygeum *(Prunus africanium)* extract in 30 patients with prostatic adenomas. The saw palmetto was superior to the pygeum in reducing symptoms, and it was much better tolerated. The *Serenoa* did not produce any side effects, while the pygeum caused gastric upset in 13 percent of the patients.

5. Bach et al. "Long-Term Drug Treatment of Benign Prostatic Hyperplasia." This 435-patient study was the first to examine the long-term activity of saw palmetto extract. There was substantial symptomatic improvement, including a 50 percent reduction in residual urine and a 6.1 milliliter per second increase in peak urinary flow rate. Eighty percent of patients and physicians rated the effects as good to very good, and *Serenoa (Sabal)* was well tolerated in 98 percent of the patients. The rate of deterioration at the end of the three-year study was significantly lower than in untreated men with BPH, which strongly suggests that long-term therapy with saw palmetto can reduce the incidence of surgery.

6. Wilt, T. et al. A recent meta-analysis of randomized controlled studies of using *Serenoa* to treat BPH was recently published in the *Journal of the American Medical Association.* The article concluded that patients and physicians rated saw palmetto as superior to the placebo and comparable to Proscar. *Serenoa* reduced nocturia by 25 percent compared to the placebo and ranked equally with Proscar at improving peak and mean urine flow rates and reducing residual urine. Side effects were comparable to the placebo and did not show the high erectile dysfunction rates associated with the use of Proscar.

ORTHODOX TREATMENTS VERSUS SAW PALMETTO FOR BPH

Pharmaceutical treatments for this common but annoying condition include finasteride (trade name: Proscar) and terazosin (trade name: Hytrin). Surgical procedures include the TURP procedure (transurethral resection of the prostate) and balloon dilation.

Saw palmetto, or better yet, saw palmetto in combination with supportive herbs and dietary changes, has multiple advantages over any of the orthodox procedures. It is the least costly treatment: A year's supply of standardized saw palmetto costs approximately $190 to $235, compared with $657 for finasteride and $5,000 for surgery. The effects of *Serenoa* equal or exceed those of either drug and it has only a very mild potential for side effects.

Problematic side effects associated with Hytrin include hypotension, syncope, dizziness, tachycardia, and vertigo; adverse reactions associated with Proscar include impotence, decreased libido, breast tenderness and enlargement, and hypersensitivity reactions such as a rash. Proscar can also cause birth defects, and pregnant women are strongly advised to avoid contact with the medication or even the sperm of a man taking this drug.

The potential for problems, physical and emotional, associated with either surgical procedure make a low-risk option such as

COMPARISON OF SAW PALMETTO VS. PROSCAR ON URINE FLOW RATE		
	SAW PALMETTO EXTRACT	PROSCAR
Initial measurement	9.53 milliliters/second	9.6 milliliters/second
After 3 months	13.15 milliliters/second	10.4 milliliters/second
After 12 months	*13.72 milliliters/second	11.2 milliliters/second
Percent of improvement	*44 percent in 12 months	16 percent in 12 months

* Estimate based on Bach and Ebeling, 1996

an herbal approach an attractive and in this case a viable option for BPH stages II and III.

A recent study by Bach, Schmitt, and Ebeling compared three prescriptive medications with a standardized saw palmetto extract. The drugs worked by two different mechanisms. Finasteride is a synthetic 5-alpha-reductase inhibitor, and the other two drugs, terazosin and alfuzosin, are alpha-1 blockers. In all important parameters, the saw palmetto was a comparable treatment with far fewer side effects. It decreased residual urine volume, reduced irritation, and increased urinary flow; 80 percent of patients rated their improved quality of life as good to very good.

EUROPEAN USE AND RESEARCH

The European use of phytomedicines for specific diseases or conditions has been well documented and researched. Much of the research done on herbal medicines over the last 50 years has been conducted by German, French, Italian, and Swiss researchers at major phytopharmaceutical companies.

The combination of a long history of herbal use with modern scientific research has given rise to the well-accepted use of "herbal drugs." Each of these medications has official status with proven uses. The German Komission E's monograph on saw palmetto is useful but is very narrowly defined in its scope of use, limiting the herb to "urination problems in benign prostatic hyperplasia Stages I and II." It states that the actions are anti-androgenic and antiexudative and that the medication relieves symptoms rather than the swelling of tissue.

European Botanical Products

Following are some examples of popular European botanical products used for prostatic enlargement:

- **Prosta capsules** (Fink): contains beta-sitosterol, saw palmetto, echinacea, and pumpkin seed.
- **Prostagutt capsules** (Schwabe): contains saw palmetto, nettle root, and aspen.
- **Saburgen** (Vogel and Weber): contains pumpkin seed, echinacea, aspen leaf, madder root, and saw palmetto.
- **Prostasan** (Dr. Arthur Vogel): contains saw palmetto (93 percent), goldenrod (3 percent), echinacea (2 percent), aspen (1.5 percent), and larkspur (0.5 percent).
- **Permixon** (Pierre Fabre Medicament): standardized 85 to 95 percent fatty sterol preparation of *Serenoa,* which is approved as an ethical drug (prescription) in 62 countries.
- **Sabal IDS 89** (Bioforce): a standardized 85 to 95 percent fatty sterol preparation, which has been extensively utilized in clinical research.

COMPANION HERBS FOR BPH

In addition to saw palmetto, many of the following herbs have been used to effectively treat BPH. Some, such as nettle root, have undergone scientific studies to confirm traditional uses. Others have been used empirically for hundreds of years for "men's problems" associated with old age. They may work better in combination than as individual herbs (simples).

Beggar Ticks (*Bidens* spp.)

This aggressive weedy plant has seeds that stick on clothes and animal hair. Herbalist Michael Moore, in his wonderful book *Medicinal Plants of the Pacific West*, says that "*Bidens* may be our best herb for benign prostatic hyperplasia" as it reduces tissue irritability in the urinary tract and rectum and helps to gradually shrink the swollen tissue. He suggests combining this herb with white sage, one of my favorite remedies for reducing prostate enlargement.

To make a tea from the dry herb, use 1 to 2 teaspoons per 8 ounces of boiling water, and steep 40 minutes. Take 4 ounces three times per day.

Cleavers (*Galium aparine*)

A common creeping climbing herb of disturbed woodlands and waste areas, cleavers can also be used as a bladder and prostate remedy. The fresh herb tincture is a nonirritating diuretic and a mild anti-inflammatory for the bladder, ureters, spermatic chord, prostate, and vas deferens. It works slowly to reduce irritation and pain and increase urinary flow. Tincture of the fresh herb is the preferred preparation, as the tea has only slight activity. The dosage of tincture is 60 to 80 drops three to four times a day.

Cleavers

Collinsonia Root / Leaf / Flower (*Collinsonia canadensis*)

Aromatic collinsonia is a preparation made from the fresh root, leaf, and flower of this herb. It is used for venous congestion and stagnation and for prostatic inflammation with a feeling of heaviness and constriction. "Minister's throat," varicose veins, hemorrhoids, and mitral valve prolapse also respond to treatment with this valuable herb. Tincture of aromatic collinsonia can be taken in doses of 20 to 30 drops four times a day.

Couch Grass (Elytrigia repens)

Couch grass is a common aggressive garden and lawn weed. A good guide to plants and weeds will help you identify it. It's nice to know that after weeding out the invasive white rhizomes, you can dry them and use the tea or tincture for urinary frequency with burning pain in the prostate or urethra.

To make a tea from the recently dried rhizome, place 2 teaspoons in 8 ounces of boiling water, decoct 10 minutes, and steep ½ hour. Take 2 to 3 cups per day. Dosage of the tincture is 40 to 60 drops four times per day.

Gravel Root (Eupatorium purpureum)

Gravel root is also called queen of the meadow or joe-pye-weed. It exhibits a specific influence on the genitourinary organs. Historically, it was believed to dissolve kidney stones, hence the

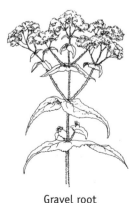

Gravel root

name gravel root. It is useful for urinary calculi or gravel, but it is not effective for diminishing kidney stones. It is, however, useful for chronic irritation of the bladder, kidney, and prostate, especially if there is pain on urination, a sensation of obstructed urinary flow, and difficult drop-by-drop passage of urine.

To make the tea, decoct 1 teaspoon of dried gravel root in 8 ounces of water for 15 minutes, then steep another ½ hour. Take 4 ounces of tea three times per day. The dosage of the tincture is 20 to 30 drops three times per day.

Horsetail (Equisitum arvense)

This plant is a descendant of the ancient tree-sized calamites, which flourished three hundred million years ago. It is used today as a tea, tincture, or capsule for BPH or prostatitis with sharp stinging pain and scanty urine of a dark color.

To make the tea, steep 1 teaspoon of the dried herb in 8 ounces of hot water for 40 to 50 minutes. Take 4 ounces three times per day. The dosage for capsules of the dried herb is 2 or 3 00 capsules per day. The dosage of the tincture is 20 to 40 drops, three times per day.

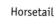
Horsetail

Hydrangea Root Bark (Hydrangea arborescens)

The wild hydrangea is a relative of the beautiful garden shrubs we are all familiar with. One of our best urinary anodynes (painkillers), it is used for urinary tract pain associated with prostatic enlargement.

To make the tea, place 1 teaspoon of the dried root bark in 8 ounces of cold water and let it steep 6 to 8 hours. Take 4 ounces, four times a day. The dosage of tincture is 20 to 40 drops four times a day.

Nettle Root (Urtica dioica)

Nettle leaf is a well-known herb. The nettle root is little known but is an effective medicine. It combines well with saw palmetto for the treatment of prostatic symptoms. Like *Serenoa*, nettle root inhibits the breakdown of testosterone into dihydrotestosterone. The mechanism for this is believed to be its inhibition of both 5-alpha-reductase and aromatase. While nettle root is less effective than saw palmetto, the two together or with pygeum have greater activity than either herb by itself.

Nettle

Pumpkin Seed Extract (Curcubita pepo)

The common pumpkin seed has been extensively studied for its beneficial effect on prostate health. Seed extracts inhibit 5-alpha-reductase conversion of testosterone to dihydrotestosterone. The mechanism of action seems to be different from that of saw palmetto, nettle root, or pygeum. Researchers speculate that beta-sitosterol (a phytosterol) competes with androgens, thus decreasing esposure of the prostate to hormonal stimulation. Eating pumpkin seeds (1 to 2 ounces per day) or taking gel capsules (2 to 4 per day) has shown benefits in reducing inflammation and other prostatic symptoms.

Pygeum Bark (Prunus africanum)

This is the bark of an evergreen tree found in Africa. Pygeum seems to work by inhibiting cholesterol uptake and antagonizing testosterone, thus reducing prostatic symptoms. It has also been found to stimulate prostatic and bulbourethral secretions. In tests comparing pygeum with *Serenoa,* pygeum was not tolerated as well, nor did it have as great an effect for relieving prostatic symptoms. The two herbs are often used together, as the mechanisms of action are somewhat different. Pygeum was found to work best with early BPH, infertility, and impotence associated with BPH or prostatitis. Pygeum is usually taken in capsule form; the daily dose is 1 to 2 100-mg capsules per day. One other important issue concerning pygeum is that it is harvested only from the wild. The supply is quite limited, and until it is commercially cultivated we should avoid regular use of this threatened species.

Small Flavored Willow Herb (Epilobium parviflorum)

Maria Treben, the well-known Austrian herbalist, highly recommended this little-known herb for kidney, bladder, and prostate disorders. Not only did she recommend it for BPH; she believed it very beneficial for prostatic cancer. In her best-selling book *Health Through God's Pharmacy,* she related two interesting case histories, one of prostate cancer and the other of bladder cancer, that she claims were successfully treated with willow herb tea.

To make the tea, use 1 to 2 teaspoons of the dried herb in 8 ounces of boiling water, and steep 30 minutes. Take 2 cups per day.

Sourwood (Oxydendrum arboreum)

The leaves of this common southeastern tree have been used in Native American, folk, and eclectic medicine for treating prostatic disease. Its indications are for chronic enlargement of the prostate, with irritation at the neck of the bladder and dysuria.

To make the tea, use 2 teaspoons of the dried leaf in 8 ounces of boiling water, let steep 30 minutes, and strain. Take 2 cups per day.

Thuja (Thuja occidentalis)

Eclectic practitioners used thuja, or flat cedar, for prostatic enlargement with dribbling of urine and frequent nocturnal urination, especially in old men. The tincture is taken in small amounts, 5 to 10 drops, two or three times per day, usually combined with other, more mild herbs. Overdoses can worsen urinary and kidney irritation.

Thuja

White Sage (Salvia apiana)

This plant is a relatively little-known member of the sage family, native to southern California. While I am unaware of any clinical studies on the activity of white sage, empirical use indicates that this herb reduces prostatic swelling, inflammation, excessive urination, and mucus discharge. It also acts as an antagonist to the hormone prolactin, which has been shown to increase prostatic

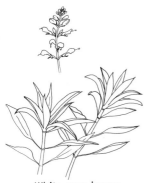

White sage leaves
and flowering top

DHT levels. Like many sages, white sage is a strong antioxidant, antibacterial, and anti-inflammatory agent. White sage tea is an intense-tasting beverage.

To make the tea, put 1 teaspoon of the dried leaf in 8 ounces of hot water, and steep covered for 20 to 30 minutes. Take 4 ounces three times per day. The tincture can be taken in doses of 20 to 30 drops three or four times per day.

Wintergreen Leaf (Gaultheria procumbens)

This plant is the source of the essential oil used in to flavor candy, toothpaste, and mouthwashes. Eclectic physicians recommended wintergreen tincture for irritation and subacute inflammation of the bladder, urethra, and prostate. Its primary action is in relieving dysuria (difficult urination), making it easier to void urine. A flavorful tea can be made with dried wintergreen leaf.

To make the tea, use 2 teaspoons of the leaf, steeped in 8 ounces of hot water (covered) for 30 minutes. A reasonable dosage is 2 cups per day.

HERBAL FORMULAS FOR PROSTATE CONDITIONS

My experience with BPH patients clearly indicates that one herb is rarely adequate to fully address the entire symptom picture. I believe that intelligently designed formulas based on clinical experience offer a wider spectrum of therapeutic activity. My formula is based on my twenty-five years of herbal practice. I strongly feel that this combination of herbs is far superior to any of the individual herbs by themselves. Dr. Clymer's formula for a related condition, prostatitis, is also based on decades of clinical experience.

David Winston's Formula for Benign Prostatic Hyperplasia

Together, the herbs in this formula are vastly more effective than any of the individual ingredients. Over the years, many patients who had limited success with only saw palmetto or pharmaceutical preparations have responded to this preparation.

Mix together tinctures of:

Aromatic collinsonia *(Collinsonia canadensis)*	1 part
Nettle root *(Urtica dioica)*	1 part
Saw palmetto *(Serenoa repens)*	1 part
White sage *(Salvia apiana)*	1 part

Suggested use: 4 milliliters (80 drops) four times per day.

Dr. R. Swinburne Clymer's Tincture Formula for Prostatitis

Dr. Clymer was a physiomedical physician who had remarkable success over a very long career treating "incurable" diseases. His book, Nature's Healing Agents, *was published in 1905 but is still in print today. This is his formula for treating prostate problems. (Note: Pasque flower is toxic in overdose. Stay within recommended dosage.)*

Mix together tinctures of:

Couch grass *(Elytrigia repens)*	5 to 15 drops
Pasque flower *(Anemone pulsatilla)*	2 to 4 drops
Pipsissewa *(Chimaphila umbellata)*	2 to 10 drops
Saw palmetto *(Serenoa repens)*	10 to 20 drops

Mix in 4 ounces of water, and take four times per day.

TRADITIONAL CHINESE MEDICINE TREATMENTS FOR BPH

In Chinese medicine, several traditional formulas are used to treat mild to moderate prostatic enlargement. Two of the most common formulas, which are available in most health food stores or from practitioners of Oriental medicine, are described here.

Rehmannia Eight Formula (Ba Wei Di Huang Wan)

This formula contains rehmannia, poria, tree peony, cinnamon, dioscorea, cornus, processed aconite, and water plantain root. It is probably the most frequently used formula for urinary problems. The herbs in the formula are anti-inflammatory, diuretic, astringent, and antibacterial. It improves the kidney, bladder, and nerve function and circulation to the urinary tract, reduces stagnation and heat, and strengthens reproductive organs such as the prostate.

Cephalanoplos Decoction (Xiao Ji Yin Zi)

This formula contains cephalanoplos (small thistle), lotus rhizome node, dry-fried cattail pollen, rehmannia, talc, mutong, lophatheri, gardenia fruit, dang gui, and honey-fried licorice. These herbs are antibacterial, anti-inflammatory, demulcent, and astringent. The formula is used for bloody, painful urinary conditions with urinary frequency and burning pain on voiding. From a Western perspective, this formula is used for acute cystitis, polycystic kidneys, kidney stones, and BPH.

DIET FOR A HEALTHY PROSTATE

Diet is a major factor in human health, and its importance to prostate health is no exception. Comparisons of the average American diet with Asian diets have revealed some interesting facts. Prostate problems, including cancer, are much less frequent in the Orient than in the United States. Japan has only one-fourth the rate of prostate cancer as the United States. When Japanese men come to U.S. and eat an American diet, their rate of prostate problems increases to match the levels of the general population. Foods that contribute to this problem include high levels of saturated fats in the diet (especially hydrogenated fats, partially hydrogenated fats, and fried foods), excessive consumption of refined carbohydrates (such as sugar, fructose, and white flour), excessive alcohol use (especially beer), and a high animal-protein diet with its added synthetic hormones.

Many foods can help keep the prostate healthy and possibly help to prevent prostatic cancer, but most are lacking in the average American diet. Soy is an important component of the Asian diet. It contains numerous compounds called isoflavones, which act as phytoestrogens, influencing prostate tissue and reducing DHT levels. Soy contains genistein and daidzein as well as other active isoflavones. Diets high in fiber also decrease the risks of bowel, prostate, and rectal cancer, and some foods such as flax seed are high in lignans — chemicals that also act as phytoestrogens.

Antioxidants play an important role in preventing cancer, and a diet rich in foods that contain antioxidants will reduce the risk of cancer and other degenerative diseases. Antioxidants that are especially beneficial to prostate health include the mineral zinc, found in pumpkin seeds, fish, seaweeds, mushrooms, nuts, and brewer's yeast. An essential but often lacking nutrient, zinc is found in high concentration in prostatic tissue. Zinc reduces prolactin levels in the blood, thereby helping inhibit the enzyme 5-alpha-reductase, and is also essential for the conversion of carotenes into Vitamin A in the body.

Vitamin A and the associated carotenoids not only reduce the risk of cancer but also strongly inhibit tissue oxidation and free radical damage. Dietary sources of Vitamin A and carotenoids include fish liver oils, dark green leafy vegetables, yellow and red vegetables, beets, spirulina, and garlic.

Vitamin B_6 is believed to help the prostate because it reduces prolactin levels and increases the absorption of zinc. Vitamin B_6 is found in brewer's yeast, peas, eggs, carrots, nuts, seeds, and fish.

Lipoic acid is a vitally important antioxidant that also aids in the recycling of other antioxidants, especially vitamins C and E, coenzyme Q_{10}, and glutathione. While it is found in meats and potatoes, adequate amounts are unlikely to be provided via food sources. Lipoic acid as a supplement helps to prevent oxidative damage associated with aging, disease, and metabolism.

Certain isolated amino acids — L-glutamine, L-alanine, and glycine — when taken together as a supplement have shown beneficial activity in reducing the symptoms of BPH.

One important group of nutrients, rarely included in the Western diet, is the essential fatty acids. These compounds are precursors to prostaglandins, which inhibit testosterone binding in the prostate. They also act as anti-inflammatory agents and restrain protein synthesis and cell growth in the prostate. The omega-3 marine lipids eicosapentaenoic acid (EPA) and docosahexaenoic acid (DHA) have been shown to inhibit the growth of prostatic tumors. Flax seed, a rich source of essential fatty acids, has been shown to inhibit cancer metastasis in studies done with mice.

Other nutrients that have a beneficial effect on the prostate include magnesium, vitamins C and E, and selenium.

PROSTATE CANCER

Thirty percent of American men over the age of 50 will develop prostate cancer. This very serious disease was once rare but now is increasingly common. In 1995, 244,000 new cases of prostate cancer were diagnosed in the United States, and there were over 40,000 fatalities from this disease. Many of the same factors that lead to BPH are linked to increased levels of prostate cancer, such as environmental pollutants, exogenous hormones, high-fat and high-calorie diets, and chronic stress.

RECOMMENDED DOSES OF NUTRIENTS TO PROMOTE PROSTATE HEALTH	
NUTRIENT	**AVERAGE DAILY DOSAGE**
Mixed carotenoids	25,000 International Units per day
Essential fatty acids (omega-3 and -6)	
Flax seed	1000 milligrams, six to nine times per day
Pumpkin or evening primrose seed oil	500 milligrams, three to six times per day
EPA / DHA	1200 milligrams, three times per day
L-glutamine, L-alanine, glycine (in combination)	Two 6-gram capsules, three times per day for 2 weeks, then one capsule three times per day.
Lipoic acid	50 milligrams, twice a day
Magnesium oxide	400 to 600 milligrams
Selenium	200 micrograms
Vitamin A	10,000 International Units
Vitamin B6	50 to 100 milligrams; take with other B vitamins
Vitamin C (ascorbate form)	250 milligrams twice a day
Vitamin E	400 to 800 International Units
Zinc picolinate	15 to 40 milligrams
Lipoic acid	50 milligrams twice per day

While there is no clinical evidence showing that saw palmetto prevents prostate cancer, increased DHT and prolactin levels have been linked to a higher incidence of this disease. Prostate cancer is stimulated by excess androgens, especially in the early stages, and orthodox therapies use treatments that suppress testosterone production. Theoretically, the use of herbs that inhibit the production of DHT and prolactin may reduce the risk of prostatic cancer and/or slow its growth. Dr. William Mitchell, N.D., a remarkable practitioner, teacher, and researcher, has stated that he believes saw palmetto to be of benefit as an anticancer agent because it blocks DHT, by inhibiting 5-alpha-reductase and 3-ketosteroid reductase. Of course, these data are theoretical and are supported by limited clinical experience.

In addition, *Serenoa* has been found to reduce cholesterol levels within prostatic tissue. This is notable because higher levels of this substance are found in prostate glands with cancer than in those without. Saw palmetto also contains an acylglyceride, 1-monolaurin, which has shown mild activity against one type of prostatic cancer cell in laboratory experiments. Hence, the use of saw palmetto, as well as nettle root *(Urtica dioica),* pygeum *(Prunus africanum),* and pumpkin seed, may offer hope and protection to our aging male population.

Other Herbs, Foods, and Supplements That May Help Prevent Prostate Cancer

Genistein and **daidzein** directly affect testosterone metabolism, reducing the toxic metabolites of testosterone. Genistein, an isoflavone, also seems to slow or prevent the metastasis of invasive cancer cells. It is believed to work by preventing the formation of new blood vessels to cancerous tumors. Histoculture studies of genistein have shown that this phytochemical reduces the growth of prostatic cancer tissue.

Fermented soy such as tempeh, miso, and tamari are healthy sources of both genistein and daidzein. Soy also contains two other antitumor compounds: beta-sitosterol and Bowman-Birk inhibitor.

Licorice *(Glycyrrhiza glabra)* is a powerful adaptogenic herb that contains genistein. It is a component of the traditional Hoxey formula, which is used to treat cancer and other chronic degenerative diseases. Licorice acts as an immune amphoteric, anti-inflammatory agent, expectorant, and Qi tonic.

Licorice

Lima beans are a rich source of genistein. Other beans and peas (especially sprouted beans), black beans, and black-eyed peas also contain this isoflavone.

Bu Gu Zhi *(Psoralea corylifolia),* a Chinese herb, is more than 60 times richer than soybeans in genistein. It is used in traditional Chinese medicine for diarrhea, frequent urination or urinary incontinence, low back pain, and wheezing.

Kudzu *(Pureria lobata)* is known as "the vine that ate the South." Yes, there are uses for this highly aggressive weed. The root is commonly used in Chinese medicine as a heart tonic, demulcent, and antispasmodic, and to reduce alcohol consumption. It also is a rich source of daidzein.

Red clover *(Trifolium pratense)* is a rich source of genistein and daidzein as well as two other important phytosterols, biochanin and formononetin. It has traditionally been used as an alterative, as a lymph and liver tonic, and to prevent and to treat various cancers.

Lycopene, a highly active carotenoid, is found in tomatoes (especially tomato sauces and ketchup), watermelon, pink grapefruit, guava, and calendula flowers. Men who regularly consume lycopene have a lower incidence of prostate cancer.

Modified citrus pectin is a nontoxic form of pectin. Animal studies published in the *Journal of the National Cancer Institute* showed that oral consumption of this substance inhibited metatasis of prostate cancer cells.

Vitamin E is a fat-soluble nutrient. A study done in Finland showed that men taking it had a reduced risk (approximately one third) of prostate cancer. In those who did have the disease, the death rate was reduced by 41 percent.

Inositol hexaphospate (IP6) is a naturally occurring compound found in corn, sesame, wheat, and rice. In human trials, this substance inhibited prostate cancer, and in laboratory studies, it caused cancer cells to revert to normal cells.

Foods That Inhibit and Prevent Cancers (Nonspecific)

Brazil nuts are an excellent source of the trace element selenium, a powerful antioxidant. On average, three Brazil nuts contain 200 micrograms of selenium, which is an effective dose for helping to reduce the possibility of carcinoma, including prostate cancer.

Grifola fungus *(Grifola frondosa)* is also known as maitake and hen of the woods. A potent immune amphoteric, it is being clinically tested for use with advanced prostate and breast cancer. A rich source of immune-potentiating high-molecular-weight polysaccharides, this medicinal mushroom shows promise for prevention of carcinomas as well as for treatment.

The omega-3 marine lipids Eicosapentaenoic acid (EPA) and docosahexaenoic acid (DHA) have been shown in studies to inhibit many types of tumors, including prostate cancer.

Brassicas, or cruciferous vegetables, are members of the mustard/cabbage family of plants (broccoli, broccoli sprouts, brussels sprouts, cabbage, cauliflower, bok choy, turnip greens, etc.). They contain chemical compounds known as indoles, which have clearly been shown to have anticancer activity as well as antibacterial, antiulcer, and antiasthmatic qualities.

Alliums are garlic, onions, scallions, shallots, ramps, leeks, and chives, which are all botanically related. Although they are usually thought of as foods, these powerful herbs contain many active sulfur compounds that have shown the ability to prevent cancer.

Green tea *(Camellia sinensis)* has long been used as a flavorful beverage throughout the world. Recent research has found that regular consumption of green tea reduces the risk of many types of cancer. Animal studies have shown that green tea may help prevent prostate cancer as well as breast, lung, stomach, and skin cancers.

6

USING SAW PALMETTO
FOR OTHER
HEALTH CONDITIONS

In this chapter we are going to explore some of the more experimental uses of saw palmetto, looking at cross-cultural analysis of the herb as well as possible medicinal applications based on theoretical data or limited clinical experience.

MALE PATTERN BALDNESS

Male pattern balding is a problem that affects the male ego and image more than physical health. The search for a cure for this adverse effect of heredity and aging has consumed a tremendous amount of time and money from ancient times until today. Ancient Egyptians anointed balding heads with the fat of a lion, a hippopotamus, a crocodile, a cat, a serpent, and an ibex to regrow hair. Today men apply Minoxidil daily to their scalps in an attempt to regrow hair. Finasteride, which has been only moderately successful in BPH, is now being sold under the trade name of Propecia as the only oral medication demonstrated to regrow hair. Finasteride works because it inhibits the enzyme 5-alpha-reductase, which, as previously mentioned, converts testosterone to dihydrotestosterone (DHT). There are several theories as to how DHT influences hair loss. One is that its absence stalls the cyclic growth of hair, preventing loss at the stage when hair is shed. If this is true, the higher the level of DHT, the greater the hair loss. Another theory suggests that DHT stimulates the sebaceous glands and sebum production, which may influence the hair cycle by impairing circulation and nutrition to the hair follicle.

A few case histories, along with our knowledge of the biochemical mechanisms that give saw palmetto and other 5-alpha-reductase inhibiting herbs their activity, suggests that an herbal approach to treating male pattern baldness may possibly exist. Saw palmetto, nettle root, pygeum bark, and pumpkin seed may have some activity for reducing or preventing hair loss. James Duke, Ph.D., an eminent economic botanist, author, and lecturer, has stated that if Propecia works then he believes saw palmetto should work as well. He also cites three anecdotal cases in which saw palmetto seemed to help stimulate new hair growth.

Other Herbs That May Help Reduce Hair Loss

Many of these herbs act as circulatory stimulants by promoting increased peripheral circulation, including circulation to the scalp, which may help improve the health of the scalp and hair and reduce balding.

Ginkgo *(Ginkgo biloba)* has shown activity in increasing peripheral and cerebral circulation. Recent studies published in the *Journal of the American Medical Association* (JAMA) showed a protective effect for ginkgo for people with Alzheimer's disease. One Japanese study (Kobayashi et al, 1993) claims that a 70 percent alcohol extract of this herb applied topically stimulated hair growth in shaved laboratory mice. No other studies have found this activity, but it does suggest a possible new use for ginkgo.

Nettle leaf *(Urtica dioica)* has a long tradition of being used for weak, unhealthy, or falling hair. The dried leaf can be made into a tea, which is used as a rinse. It is used to nourish the hair, reduce sebum production on the scalp, and reduce hair loss.

Bacopa monneria has been shown in recent studies to stimulate hair growth in laboratory mice. Traditionally, this Ayurvedic herb, known as brahmi, was used to increase hair growth, stimulate cerebral circulation, and treat impaired memory and poor concentration.

Rosemary (*Rosmarinus officinalis*) has long been used as a hair wash. This aromatic spice improves circulation to the scalp, removes dandruff and sebum accumulations and leaves the hair clean, fragrant, and shiny.

Horse chestnut (*Aesculus hippocastanum*) is a source of esculine, an extract from the common horse chestnut seed. Along with ximenynic and lauric acids, esculin has markedly reduced hair loss in male pattern balding. The preparation has improved scalp circulation, reduced seborrhea, and improved the hair's vitality.

Gu Sui Bu/Drynaria rhizome is used topically in traditional Chinese medicine to stimulate hair growth and to treat baldness.

POLYCYSTIC OVARY DISEASE

Polycystic ovary disease (Stein-Leventhal syndrome) is a increasingly common condition affecting young to middle-aged women. The symptoms can include amenorrhea, hirsutism, obesity, enlarged ovaries, irregular menses with profuse bleeding, and multiple ovarian cysts. The condition usually appears after puberty and gradually worsens over time. The cause of this benign but problematic condition is believed to be a functional derangement of hormonal secretions. Androgen and luteinizing levels tend to be elevated, while follicle-stimulating hormone levels are usually low. Orthodox medicine has little to offer women with this disturbing condition.

Case Histories

Since saw palmetto has an anti-androgen effort, it has been suggested as a possible treatment for polycystic ovary disease. Jill

Stansbury, N.D., is the chair of the Botanical Medicine Department at the National College of Naturopathic Medicine in Portland, Oregon. In addition to her busy teaching schedule, she maintains a thriving clinical practice in Battle Ground, Washington. Her written work is frequently found in professional journals, and she is the author of *Herbs for Health and Healing*. Dr. Stansbury has shared two successful case histories of polycystic ovary disease that included *Serenoa* as part of the overall treatment protocol.

Case 1. A 22-year old woman came in with a chief complaint of amenorrhea. She reported a rather late menarche at the age of 17. She had had regular cycles for a only a few months, with heavy cramping and menstrual flow; then her cycles became increasingly erratic and stopped altogether when she was about 18. She tried birth control pills for over three years, switching to different types and strengths, but none were effective in inducing regular cycles.

The patient was otherwise very healthy. She reported no other health problems, a review of her body systems showed no abnormalities, and she was rarely ill. Blood samples were taken at the first appointment, and her blood counts and blood chemistry were normal. The levels of follicle-stimulating hormone and luteinizing hormone were in normal ranges, but the serum testosterone was significantly elevated. Follow-up ultrasonography revealed several small cysts on each ovary, confirming the diagnosis of polycystic ovary disease.

We began a formula of equal parts of *Vitex, Angelica,* and *Serenoa* in a ratio of 1:1 and 1:2 tinctures, at a dosage of ½ teaspoon three times a day. The patient had a menstrual period 3 weeks after starting the formula. Menses began occurring every 4 to 6 weeks, and the formula was refilled many times over the following year. She stopped the formula for several months while traveling in Mexico and became amenorrheic again. Once she was home and resumed taking the formula, menses resumed. She has continued to have regular menses for over five years now.

Case 2. A 32-year-old married woman came in with a chief complaint of infertility and a complex gynecologic history including sexual abuse in childhood, several episodes of pelvic inflammatory disease, multiple ovarian cysts, and intermittent periods of amenorrhea. She and her husband wished to conceive but were unsuccessful after two years of unprotected intercourse.

The patient was basically amenorrheic, having only 1 or 2 menses a year. She also experienced mild constipation, frequent gas and bloating, acne, and increasing facial hair. Oral contraceptives had been used in the past and were effective in inducing regular menstrual cycles, but amenorrhea returned as soon as they were discontinued. Birth control pills also made the acne and digestive complaints worse and obviously were not an option for promoting fertility.

The results of pelvic examination and blood chemistry tests were entirely normal. The levels of follicle-stimulating hormone and luteinizing hormone were normal, while serum testosterone was elevated. Pelvic ultrasonography revealed multiple cysts on each ovary.

We formulated an herbal tea made with dandelion root, yellow dock root, Oregon grape root, burdock root, licorice root, fennel seed, cinnamon bark, and citrus peel, of which she drank 2 to 3 cups per day. We also made a tincture formula with equal parts of *Vitex, Serenoa,* and *Dioscorea,* which was to be taken ½ teaspoon three times a day.

After one month, she had less gas and improved digestion, her acne was diminishing, with fewer new breakouts, and she had no menses. After two months, her digestion and complexion continued to improve, and menses had occurred the previous week. At her three-month and six-month checkups, she was having regular monthly menses. By eight months, her menses were regular, but she had still not conceived. At her 12-month checkup, she was two months pregnant. Unfortunately, she experienced a miscarriage at 11 weeks of pregnancy. The miscarriage was not related to the herbs, without which she wouldn't likely have conceived.

Continued treatment and tonification of the uterus might have been successful in helping to achieve and bring a second pregnancy to term, but the patient moved and has since been lost to follow up.

Other Herbs for Polycystic Ovarian Disease

The berries (fruits) of the Mediterranean chaste tree (*Vitex agnus-castus*) are used for a wide range of female reproductive imbalances. Chaste tree works via the pituitary gland, helping balance the levels of follicle-stimulating hormone and luteinizing hormone, thus normalizing the ratios of progesterone, estrogen, and androgen. *Vitex* combined with *Serenoa* and liver-clearing herbs such as dandelion root, yellow dock root, or Oregon grape root has been successful in treating polycystic ovary disease.

Formulas for Ovarian Pain and Infertility

Eclectic use of *Serenoa* clearly showed that this herb is also useful for ovarian pain such as mittelschmerz or pain caused by ovarian cysts. The following formula is one that I have used with patients many times with good success.

Women's Tincture Formula for Ovarian Pain or Ovarian Cysts

Mix together tinctures of:

Blue cohosh (*Caulophyllum thalictroides*)	1 part
Chaste tree (*Vitex agnus-castus*)	2 parts
Corydalis (*Corydalis yanhusuo*)	1 part
Dan shen (*Salvia miltiorrhiza*)	2 parts
Saw palmetto (*Serenoa repens*)	2 parts

Suggested use: 4 milliliters (80 drops) three times a day.

Tincture Formula for Infertility (Women)

Mix together tinctures of:

Chaste tree *(Vitex agnus-castus)*	2 parts
Helonias *(Chaemilirium luteum)*	1 part
Saw palmetto *(Serenoa repens)*	2 parts
Shatavari *(Asparagus racemosus)*	2 parts

Suggested use: 3 milliliters (60 drops) three or four times per day.

Also take essential fatty acids (3–4 grams), especially omega-3, and vitamin E (400 International Units) daily.

In chapter 3, I discussed a case of male infertility in which saw palmetto was noted. The formula below is designed to treat female infertility associated with elevated androgen, elevated estrogen, and low progesterone levels.

DEEP CYSTIC ACNE

Deep cystic acne is a complex condition that involves an interaction between hormones (testosterone), sebum, and bacteria. It starts at puberty when the increase in androgen levels causes greater activity of the sebaceous glands. This leads to increased growth of epidermal tissue, which blocks the follicle and creates a comedo (cyst) composed of sebum, keratin, and bacteria. Irritation of the follicular wall follows, with rupture of the follicle and then an acute inflammatory reaction. This leads to an abscess and finally healing with scar tissue.

Saw palmetto may be of benefit for this condition because of its binding effects on androgens. Better yet, a combination of

Serenoa with Oregon grape root, alder bark, and chaste tree has shown clinical activity in helping to control and alleviate this disfiguring condition. Long-term use has led to reduced formation of cysts and the resultant scarring.

Other Herbs for Cystic Acne

Alder bark *(Alnus serrulata, A. rubra).* The eclectic indications for alder bark are skin conditions with pustular eruptions, weakened vitality, and constipation.

To make a tea, put 1 teaspoon of the dried bark in 8 ounces of boiling water and steep for 40 minutes. Take 4 ounces of the tea three or four times per day. As a tincture the dosage is 30 to 40 drops, three or four times per day.

Oregon grape root *(Mahonia aquafolium).* This is one of the preeminent skin/acne remedies of the eclectic physicians. It is used for a wide array of skin problems, especially chronic ones involving liver congestion and a slight yellow hue to the skin. It can also be used topically as a wash for acne and acne rosacea.

To make the intensely bitter tea, decoct 1 teaspoon of the dried root bark in 8 ounces of water for 15 minutes, then steep it for another 45 minutes. The dosage is 4 ounces of the tea, three times per day. The tincture dose is 30 to 50 drops (1 to 2 milliliters) three times per day.

Chaste tree *(Vitex agnus-castus).* Chaste tree has shown activity for hormonally induced acne, especially when it is exacerbated in association with the menstrual cycle.

Topical Herbal Applications for Acne

Gotu kola *(Centella asiatica).* A common herb of Southeast Asia, this creeping plant has been used for thousands of years in Ayurvedic medicine. Traditionally, it has been used as a diuretic, a cerebral tonic, and a treatment for leprosy as well as for inflammatory skin and muscle conditions. It is applied topically as a

David Winston's Tincture Formula for Deep Cystic Acne

Mix together tinctures of:

Chaste tree *(Vitex agnus-castus)*	2 parts
Saw palmetto *(Serenoa repens)*	2 parts
Oregon grape root *(Mahonia aquafolium)*	1 part
Sarsaparilla (*Smilax* spp.)	1 part
Red alder bark *(Alnus serrulata)*	1 part

Suggested use: 4 to 5 milliliters (80 to 100 drops) three times per day.

Also, take B complex vitamins (25 milligrams twice per day) and omega-3 fatty acids (3–4 grams daily).

poultice or ointment to speed the healing of skin tissue, to relieve inflammation, and to help prevent scarring. It can be used externally for acne, burns, and psoriasis.

CHINESE PERSPECTIVES ON USING SAW PALMETTO

There is a common thread in the literature concerning the use of saw palmetto. Early observers noticed animals that were thin and poorly nourished gained weight and strength after eating saw palmetto. Early physicians noted its use for anorexia, asthenic depletion, sexual neurasthenia, atrophy of sexual organs, lung weakness, loss of libido, and infertility. These uses are consistent with the use of what in Chinese medicine are known as the harmony remedies. Although saw palmetto is not used in traditional Chinese medicine, we can examine its activity using principles and concepts from that branch of medical practice.

A Traditional Chinese Medicine Perspective

The taste of the berries is sweet and acrid; the energy is warm and moist (oily). The taste, the energy, and the plant's activity tell us that saw palmetto fits into the category of herbs known as Qi tonics. It would be a superior or kingly remedy used to tonify, nourish, and strengthen the Chinese organs known as the Lungs, Spleen, and Kidney (which do not necessarily correspond to the organs as they are described in Western anatomy and medicine).

In Chinese medicine, the Lungs not only take in air but extract from it the vital essence known as Air Qi. This is combined in the lungs with Grain Qi to create Xue (Blood) and the protective Wei Qi. Thus, in Chinese medicine the Lungs bring in oxygen, help create the Blood, and maintain an energy field that protects us from external pernicious influences (cold, heat, dampness, dryness, wind, etc.). From a Western perspective, this can be associated with increased macrophage and immune activity, preventing illness from colds, flu, and allergies caused by bacteria, virus, and fungi.

The Chinese Spleen is responsible, among other activities, for absorbing the vital essence of food, the Grain Qi. Spleen Qi tonics increase nutrition and vitality, and they contribute to creating Blood. The Spleen also helps to keep Blood in its proper channels and maintains the Upright Qi, which prevents organ prolapse and helps with fluid metabolism.

The Chinese Kidney not only controls fluid metabolism but also stores Jing, or the life force, the primal essence. Without Jing there is no life, no growth, no maturation, no sexual activity or procreation. The Chinese Kidneys control reproductive functions and certain endocrine functions (especially adrenal activity), and, as previously mentioned, governs fluid metabolism.

Once we understand the Chinese classifications and compare the Western uses of this remarkable herb, it becomes clear that saw palmetto is a Western version of the much better-known Chinese adaptogenic remedies such as Chinese ginseng, codonopsis, prince seng, American ginseng, and licorice.

Adaptogens are remedies that normalize functions throughout the body, primarily by affecting the endocrine, immune, and nervous systems. They increase our resistance to stress, strengthen immune potential, and nourish and normalize tissue (reproductive, digestive, respiratory). Saw palmetto has all of these activities and more, as it also removes dampness and stagnation from the Lower Jiao (part of the Chinese "organ" system which incorporates the Kidney, Spleen, and Lungs).

Formulas to Reduce Stress and Strengthen the Immune System

The following formulas are combinations of Chinese herbs, saw palmetto, and Western herbs.

David Winston's Immune Reservoir Formula

This immune formula is a Fu Zheng remedy used to strengthen immune potential, adrenal/hypothalamus function, reduce histamine response (allergies), and tonify the Chinese Spleen.

Mix together tinctures of:

Astragalus *(Astragalus membranaceus)*	1 part
Ganoderma *(Ganoderma sinensis, Ganoderma lucidum)*	1 part
Saw palmetto *(Serenoa repens)*	1 part
Siberian ginseng *(Eleutherococcus senticosis)*	1 part

Suggested use: Take 5 milliliters (1 teaspoon) three times a day.
To make a tea: Place 2 teaspoons of dried herbs in 16 ounces of hot water. Decoct slowly for 1 hour. Reduce liquid by half, to 8 ounces. Take 2 or 3 cups of the tea per day.

Formula for Weak or Deficient Lungs

This formula is designed to strengthen deficient Lung Qi. It is useful for dry, deficient asthma, for people who regularly get lung infections and chest colds, and for emphysema and dry irritative coughs.

Mix together teas or tinctures of:

Astragalus *(Astragalus membranaceus)*	1 part
Prince seng *(Pseudostellaria heterophylla)*	1 part
Saw palmetto *(Serenoa repens)*	1 part
Sweet cicily *(Osmorrhiza* spp.)	1 part

Suggested use: Take 4 milliliters (80 drops) 3 times a day.
To make a tea: Place 2 teaspoons of the herbs in 16 ounces of hot water. Decoct slowly for 1 hour. Reduce liquid by half, to 8 ounces. Take 2 cups of the tea per day.

Also increase mixed carotenoids in the diet by eating winter squash, pumpkin, sweet and hot red or yellow peppers, sweet potatoes, apricots, beets, nettles, and garlic. Breathing exercises such as yogic breathing or Qi Gong are also helpful.

Tincture or Tea Formula for Anorexia and Asthenia

This formula combines herbs that strengthen the lungs, Chinese Spleen, and Chinese Kidney. It also builds Blood (Xue) and increases energy, endocrine function, and immune response. It is appropriate for weak, deficient people, especially those with anorexia or anemia, and for thin, tired, asthenic vegans.

Saw palmetto *(Serenoa repens)*	2 parts
American ginseng *(Panax quinquefolium)**	2 parts
Fenugreek seed *(Trigonella foenum-graecum)*	2 parts
Processed rehmania *(Rehmania glutinosa)*	1 part
Prince seng *(Pseudostellaria heterophylla)*	1 part

Suggested use: Take 3 to 5 milliliters three times per day.
To make a tea: Place 2 teaspoons of the herbs in 16 ounces of hot water. Decoct slowly for 30 minutes, or until reduced by half, and then let steep an additional 30 minutes. Take 4 ounces of the tea four times per day. Also take "super foods" such as spirulina, nettles, wheat grass powder, and royal jelly.

*Use organically woods-grown roots; avoid wildcrafted ginseng, as it is an endangered species.

Tincture Formula for Infertility (Men) and Impotence

This formula is appropriate for men who have deficient kidney yang conditions (impotence, low sperm count, low back pain, little or no libido). It combines kidney yin and yang tonics, nervines, and blood tonics to create a nourishing formula that gradually strengthens the reproductive, endocrine, and nervous systems.

Mix together tinctures of:

Dodder seed (*Cuscuta* spp.)	2 parts
Fresh oat ex *(Avena sativa)*	2 parts
He Shou Wu *(Polygonum multiflorum)*	2 parts
Sao Yang or Rou Cong Rong (*Orobanche* spp.)	1 part
Saw palmetto *(Serenoa repens)*	2 parts

Suggested use: Take 5 milliliters (1 teaspoon) three times per day.

Also take zinc (20 to 30 milligrams per day) and essential fatty acids, especially omega-3 (3–4 grams per day).

AYURVEDIC PERSPECTIVE ON SAW PALMETTO

I am not trained in Ayurveda, India's ancient system of medicine, but I thought it would be interesting to compare an Ayurvedic view of *Serenoa* (although Ayurveda practitioners do not use this herb) with the traditional Chinese medicine and Western views. I invited a noted scholar of this medical system, Allan Tillotson, M.A., AHG, to do this analysis. According to Allan, "Saw palmetto fruit would be considered sweet and slightly pungent in taste. It is oily, warming in *virya* (energy), and diuretic. It reduces *pitta* (heat) and *vata* (dryness). It nourishes and relaxes the internal organs, and reduces inflammation. It strengthens *apana vayu,* thus increasing downward movement of energy so that inflammation and excess fluids can be flushed from the lung, urinary, and reproductive systems. Its *prabhava* (special power) is relaxing and reduces swelling in the prostate."

THE BRITISH EXPERIENCE WITH SAW PALMETTO

English herbalists became acquainted with the use of *Serenoa* during the early twentieth century. Prominent herbal authors such as Mrs. Leyel and Mrs. Grieve, as well as those writing in the orthodox pharmaceutical literature, served to introduce this new botanical medicine to Great Britain. British herbal practitioners have preserved the knowledge of saw palmetto's wider scope of use that has mostly been lost here in the United States. While most American herbalists consider *Serenoa* a prostate herb, we find other uses in current texts from Great Britain. The *British Herbal Pharmacopoeia* mentions three herbal combinations containing saw palmetto. The first for general debility and cachexia, contains equal parts damiana *(Turnera diffusa),* cola nut *(Cola nitida),* and saw palmetto. The second, for prostatic hypertrophy, combines horsetail, hydrangea, and saw palmetto. The last, for irritation of the genitourinary tract, has two less common herbs: pellitory-of-the-wall *(Parietaria diffusa)* and buchu *(Agathosma betulina)* mixed with the saw palmetto.

In a 1951 article in the British periodical *Health from Herbs Magazine and the Medical Herbalist,* A. Barker, MNIMH, president of the National Institute of Medical Herbalists, noted the uses of saw palmetto. Most unusual was his recommendation of using *Serenoa* not only orally but as a rectal suppository for prostate problems of older men.

In her excellent book *The Complete Women's Herbal,* British herbalist Ann McIntyre, MNIMH, not only lists the well-known uses of this herb but mentions its usefulness for "increasing milk flow in nursing mothers," for salpingitis, for nourishing patients with wasting diseases, and to regulate the menstrual cycle.

Thomas Bartram, in his recent text *Encyclopedia of Herbal Medicine,* lists *Serenoa* as an adaptogen, urinary antiseptic, tonic nutrient, endocrine stimulant, and anticatarrhal agent. He recommends the berries for a wide range of uses, not just the common urinary and prostate problems.

OTHER CONDITIONS THAT MAY BENEFIT FROM SAW PALMETTO

We have seen how saw palmetto is much more than a "prostate herb." Historical and clinical use clearly shows a wide range of uses for *Serenoa.* I don't believe we currently are aware of the full scope of the therapeutic benefits that saw palmetto possesses. As mentioned previously, there are tantalizing possibilities for the use of this herb for problems ranging from prostate cancer to male pattern balding. In other equally difficult conditions, *Serenoa* may provide some benefit as part of a complete treatment protocol.

Hypoprolactinemia is a hormonal imbalance with elevated levels of prolactin. Prolactin is normally elevated in nursing mothers, but abnormal amounts can cause impotence in men and amenorrhea and secretion of breast milk in women. A physician must first rule out the presence of a prolactinoma (pituitary tumor), but if there is no such tumor, saw palmetto along with white sage *(Salvia apiana)* and chaste tree *(Vitex agnus-castus)* may be of benefit.

Paul Barney, M.D., a physician from Layton, Utah, combines the use of orthodox medicine with herbs, nutrition, and acupuncture. At the 1998 International Saw Palmetto Symposium, he spoke of using *Serenoa* for pelvic congestion syndrome. This condition is difficult to treat; its symptoms include an engorged (boggy) uterus with feelings of heaviness, chronic pain often worse during menses, frequent urination, and painful sexual intercourse. Dr. Barney referred to a study done at the University of Buenos Aires by Professor Juan Dillon. In this study, 60 women, aged 18 to 45, were divided into three groups. Twenty women received a placebo, 20 received prescription anti-inflammatory agents, and the remaining 20 were treated with a mixture of saw palmetto and pygeum. The results were quite interesting. In the first (control) group, 20 percent of the women improved; in the second group, 50 percent improved. The women taking the herbal combination had an improvement rate of 95 percent. The preferred treatment should seem obvious.

Dr. Barney also believes that saw palmetto may be useful for treating asthma, as its anti-inflammatory properties reduce the production of inflammatory leucotrenes and prostaglandins.

CONVERTING TO METRIC MEASUREMENTS

TEASPOONS TO MILLILITERS

¼ teaspoon = 1 ml

⅓ teaspoon = 2 ml

½ teaspoon = 2.5 ml

¾ teaspoon = 4 ml

1 teaspoon = 5 ml

TABLESPOONS TO MILLILITERS

¼ tablespoon = 4 ml

½ tablespoon = 8 ml

1 tablespoon = 15 ml

CUPS TO MILLILITERS

⅛ cup = 30 ml

¼ cup = 59 ml

⅓ cup = 79 ml

½ cup = 118 ml

⅔ cup = 150 ml

¾ cup = 180 ml

1 cup = 237 ml

2 cups = 473 ml = 1 pint

4 cups = 1 quart = 946 ml, or approximately 1 liter

4 quarts = 1 gallon = 4 liters

OUNCES TO GRAMS

¼ ounce = 7 g

⅓ ounce = 9.3 g

½ ounce = 14 g

1 ounce = 28 g

2 ounces = 56 g

3 ounces = 84 g

4 ounces = 112 g

6 ounces = 168 g

8 ounces = 224 g

16 ounces = 1 pound = 454 g

2.2 pounds = 1 kilogram

INCHES TO CENTIMETERS

1 inch = 2.5 cm

GLOSSARY

Adaptogen: a nontoxic substance that helps an organism adapt to physiologic or psychologic stress. Adaptogens help normalize endocrine, immune, and nervous system functions.

Adenoma: a growth or tumor of glandular epithelum.

AHG: the American Herbalists Guild; used to denote peer-reviewed professional members of the guild.

Alopecia: absence or loss of hair, usually of the head and/or eyebrows.

Alterative: a substance that increases elimination of systemic wastes via the major eliminatory organs, including the liver, lungs, lymph, kidneys, large intestine, and skin.

Amenorrhea: lack of a menstrual cycle.

Amphoteric: a substance that normalizes function, usually via nutrition.

Anabolic agent: a steroid hormone that has testosterogenic activity and increases anabolism.

Analgesic: a substance that relieves pain.

Anodyne: a painkiller or analgesic.

Antiandrogenic: a substance that inhibits the action of androgens (testosterone).

Antigen: a protein marker on the surface of a cell that identifies that cell as belonging to that tissue (kidney, liver, etc.) or to the organism.

Antihepatotoxin: a substance that protects the liver against damage caused by poisons or viruses.

Antihistamine: a substance that reduces histamine production, thus reducing swelling and inflammation.

Antiphlogistic: anti-inflammatory.

Antiseptic: a substance that inhibits or prevents the formation of bacteria that cause sepsis (infection).

Apana Vayu: the energy governing downward movement of feces, urine, semen, menstrual fluid, and birthing.

Antiandrogenic: an inhibitor of androgen uptake or activity.

Aphonia: inability to talk; can occur with chronic laryngitis.

Ayurvedic medicine: the traditional medical system of India; *ayurveda* means "science of life."

Benign prostatic hyperplasia: a progressive condition in older men wherein the prostatic tissue swells, causing impaired urinary flow.

Borborygmus: loud intestinal rumbling or gurgling caused by passage of gas.

BPH: benign prostatic hyperplasia.

Bright's disease: nonspecific name for degenerative kidney disease.

Bulbourethral (Cowper's) glands: two small pea-sized glands on either side of the prostate. They secrete a viscous fluid that makes up part of the seminal fluid.

Cachexia: a wasting condition associated with cancer, AIDS, and tuberculosis. Patients are malnourished, fatigued, weak, and debilitated.

Carotenoid: a group of yellow, orange, and red pigments found in plant and animal tissues. Some carotenoids, such as beta-carotene, lutein, and lycopene, have antioxidant properties.

Catarrh: inflammation of a mucous membrane, with discharge of mucus or phlegm.

Chinese Kidney: the Kidneys store Jing, the vital essence; hence, they are responsible for maturation, reproduction, and development. The Kidneys also regulate water circulation, warm the body, and nourish the bone, teeth, and marrow.

Chinese Lung: the Lungs maintain respiration, taking in the Air Qi. They circulate fluids and Qi to the skin, promoting sweating and providing the Wei Qi (protective Qi).

Chinese Spleen: the Spleen is responsible for digestion and transportation of food (Grain Qi) and helping with fluid metabolism. The spleen also maintains the Upright Qi, keeps the blood within the blood vessels, and nourishes the flesh and limbs. The essence of the Grain Qi rises to the lung, where in mixing with the Air Qi it becomes Blood (Xue).

C.N.: certified nutritionist.

Decoction: a method of making tea that slowly simmers the herbs. Usually used for dense roots, seeds, and fruits.

Demulcent: a substance that is soothing and anti-inflammatory to the mucus membranes. Herbal demulcents include slippery elm bark and marsh mallow root.

DHT: Dihydrotestosterone.

Dihydrotestosterone: a potent androgen believed to stimulate the growth of prostatic tissue.

Diterpenes: bitter-tasting terpeniod compounds responsible for digestive activity in bitters and antiviral activity in mints.

Diuretic: a substance that increases urinary output. Most diuretics can be divided into two groups: irritating diuretics (juniper, cubebs) and nonirritating (corn silk, pipsissewa).

Drupe: a fleshy fruit with a soft outer part covering a hard shell that contains the seed(s).

Dysmenorrhea: menstrual pain.

Dysuria: painful or difficult urination.

Eclectic medicine: a system of medicine that emphasizes the use of medicines (mostly herbal) based on their specific actions for specific symptoms.

Emetic: a susbstance that induces vomiting.

Enuresis: involuntary urination, as in bedwetting.

Epididymitis: inflammation of the epididymis, a tube connected to the testicles.

Estradiol: one of the three forms of estrogens.

Expectorant: a substance that stimulates excretion of mucus from the lungs.

Flavonoid: a large group of compounds commonly found in plants that gives color to flowers and some leaves and roots, such as ginkgo leaf, blueberries, hibiscus flowers, and milk thistle seeds. They act as antioxidants and anti-inflammatory agents.

Follicle-stimulating hormone: a hormone produced by the pituitary that stimulates growth of the ovarian follicle and estrogen secretion.

FSH: follicle-stimulating hormone.

Hematuria: blood in the urine.

Hirsutism: excess hair on the face or body.

Histoculture: tissue culture.

Homeopathy: a system of medicine founded by Samuel Hahnemann, which has two main theoretical tenets: (1) like cures like (the law of similars) and (2) the more dilute (potentized) the remedy, the more powerful it becomes.

Hypocholesterolemic: a substance that lowers levels of cholesterol in the blood.

Ibex: a horned antelope from northern Africa and the Arabian peninsula.

Interstitial cystitis: chronic cystitis without a known bacterial cause.

Jing: vital essence, or life force. Jing is stored in the Chinese Kidney and is responsible for growth, maturation, sexuality, and reproduction.

Kapha: in Ayurvedic medicine, the water and earth humor. Kapha qualities include cold, wet, slow, and dense.

Komission E: a German regulatory agency.

L.Ac.: licensed acupuncturist.

LH: luteinizing hormone.

Lignans: widely occuring compounds that are closely related to lignan, which forms the woody part of trees and plants.

Luteinizing hormone: a hormone produced by the pituitary that in women stimulates the follicle to release a ripened ovum; in men, LH stimulates the production of testosterone and sperm cells.

Micturation: the process of urination.

Mitral valve prolapse: mild prolapse of the mitral (bicuspid) valve of the heart is common and occurs in approximately 11 percent of the population. More serious is mitral regurgitation, which allows blood from the left ventricle to backflow into the left atrium because of incomplete closure of the valve.

MNIMH: a professional member of the British National Institute of Medical Herbalists.

Mucopurulent: a discharge containing mucus and pus.

N.D.: naturopathic doctor.

Neurasthenia: nerve weakness, similar to today's chronic fatigue syndrome.

Nocturia: excessive urination during the night.

Orchitis: inflammation of the testicles caused by trauma, infection, mumps, etc.

Otitis media: an infection of the middle ear, symptomized by excess fluid and pain.

Ozena: nasal disease characterized by a profuse discharge with a fetid odor.

Palmate: fan-shaped.

Palmetto scrubs: dense colonies of saw palmetto plants.

Panicle: a compound form of flower having the younger flowers at the top of the center.

Peritonitis: inflammation of the peritoneum, the membrane that lines the abdomen.

Pertussis: whooping cough.

Pitta: in Ayurvedic medicine, the fire humor. Pitta qualities include heat, quickness, and softness.

Pollakiuria: abnormally frequent urination.

Phytoestrogens (phytosterols): compounds with very mild hormonal activity, such as licorice, red clover, and alfalfa.

Polysaccharides (glycans): compounds of high molecular weight made of chains of sugars, such as ganoderma, saw palmetto, and astragalus.

Prolactin: a hormone produced by the pituitary; among other effects, it stimulates milk production during pregnancy.

Protocol: the specific treatments used for a patient or to treat a disease.

Prostatism: another term for benign prostatic hyperplasia.

PSA: prostate specific antigen.

Puerperal fever: sepsis following childbirth; also known as childbirth fever.

Qi: energy in motion (i.e. kinetic energy). Energy that moves blood, causes respiration, and keeps the heart beating. There are many different forms of Qi; some are Wei Qi, Zhang Qi, and Grain Qi.

Salpingitis: inflammation of the fallopian tube.

Sesquiterpenes: plant chemicals usually found with essential oils. They may have evolved to protect plants from insect damage.

Spadices: plural of spadix, a spike with a thick, fleshy axis.

Sterols (phytosterols): part of a plant's cell membrane, which can have a mild amphoteric activity on human hormonal systems.

Syncope: fainting caused by inadequate blood supply to the brain.

Tachycardia: abnormally fast heartbeat (over 100 beats per minute).

Tannin: an acid phytochemical found in most tree barks. Tannins act as astringents, reducing secretions.

Tincture: a hydryalcoholic extract of herbs.

TMJ: temporomandibular joint dysfuntion.

Topical application: topical or local applications are applied externally to the skin; they include poultices, ointments, liniments, and baths.

Trabecula: a band of connective tissue.

Uremia: toxicity of the blood caused by elevated levels of nitrogen compounds normally excreted via the kidney. Often associated with renal insufficiency or severe blockage of the urinary apparatus.

Vata: in Ayurvedic medicine, the air humor. Vata qualities include dryness, cooling, hardness, and changeability.

Virya: the energetic quality of a substance, such as warming or cooling.

Wei Qi: protective energy generated by the Chinese Lungs. It is associated with the skin and protects the body from external pernicious influences (cold, heat, dampness, dryness, wind, summer heat).

Xue: in traditional Chinese medicine *xue* is translated as Blood. This is not exactly the substance we call blood in the West. Xue carries nutrition throughout the body and also lubricates the joints and muscles.

SELECTED BIBLIOGRAPHY

American Institute of Homeopathy. *The Homeopathic Pharmacopoeia of the United States.* Falls Church, VA: 1979.

American Pharmaceutical Association. *Proceedings of the American Pharmaceutical Association,* vol. 27. Baltimore: American Pharmaceutical Association, 1879.

American Pharmaceutical Association. *Proceedings of the American Pharmaceutical Association,* vol. 42. Baltimore: American Pharmaceutical Association, 1894.

American Pharmaceutical Association. *Proceedings of the American Pharmaceutical Association,* vol. 44. Baltimore: American Pharmaceutical Association, 1896.

Anonymous. *An Epitome of Therapeutics.* Philadelphia: John Wyeth and Brother Inc., 1901.

Anonymous. *British Herbal Pharmacopoeia Part II.* West Yorks, Great Britain: 1979.

Anonymous. *Fibre-Bearing Plants of Florida.* Tallahassee, FL: Department of Agriculture, 1938.

Anonymous. *Physicians Desk Reference,* 51st ed. Montvale, NJ: Medical Economics Company, 1997.

Anonymous. *The Pharmacology of the Newer Materia Medica.* Detroit, MI: G.S. Davis, 1892.

Bach, D. and L. Ebeling. "Long-Term Drug Treatment of Benign Prostatic Hyperplasia: Results of a Three-Year Multicenter Study." *Phytomedicine* 3(2): 1996, 105–111.

Bach, D., M. Schmitt, and L. Ebeling. "Phytopharmaceutical and Synthetic Agents in the Treatment of Benign Prostatic Hyperplasia (BPH)." *Phytomedicine* 3(4):1996.

Balick, M.J., Ph.D. and H.T. Beck, eds. *Useful Palms of the World.* New York: Columbia University Press, 1990.

Bartram, T. *Encyclopedia of Herbal Medicine.* Dorset, England: Grace Publishing, 1995.

Bennett, B.C., and J.R. Hicklin. "Uses of Saw Palmetto (Serenoa repens, Arecaceae) in Florida." *Economic Botany* 52(4):1998, 381–393.

Bensky, D., and R. Barolet. *Chinese Herbal Medicine-Formulas and Strategies.* Seattle: Eastland Press, 1990.

Bensky, D., and A. Gamble. *Chinese Herbal Medicine-Materia Medica.* Seattle: Eastland Press, 1986.

Berkon, R., ed. *The Merck Manual of Diagnosis & Therapy.* Rahway, NJ: Merck Research Laboratories, 1992.

Boik, J. *Cancer and Natural Medicine.* Princeton, MN: Oregon Medical Press, 1996.

Bombardelli, E., and P. Morazzoni. *Prunus Afraicana.* Hook F. Kalkim, *Fitoterapia* 68(3): 205–218, 1997.

Bombardelli, E., and P. Morazzoni. *Serenoa Repens (Bartram). Fitoterapia* 68(2): 99–114, 1997.

Bone, K. "Saw Palmetto — A Critical Review." *The European Journal of Herbal Medicine* 4(1): 15–24, 1998.

Braeckman, J. "The Extract of *Serenoa repens* in the Treatment of Benign Prostatic Hyperplasia." *Current Therapeutic Research* 55: 776–85, 1994.

Braeckman, J., and J. Bruhwyler., et al. "Efficacy and Safety of the Extract of Serenoa repens in the Treatment of Benign Prostatis Hyperplasia: Therapeutic Equivalence between Twice and Once Daily Dosage Forms." *Phytotherapy Research,* 11: 558–563, 1997.

Brue, W., and M. Hagenlocher, et al. "Antiphlogistic Activity of an Extract from Sabal [sic] serrulata Fruits Prepared by Supercritical Carbon Dioxide." *Arzneim-Forsch Drug Report* 42: 547–51, 1992.

Brodie, William, M.D., ed. *New Preparations,* vol. 3, no. 7. Detroit, MI: 1879.

Burlage, H. *Index of Plants of Texas with Reputed Medicinal and Poisonous Properties.* Austin, Texas: Burlage, 1968.

Champault et al. "Medical treatment of Prostatic Adenoma." *Ann Lerol* (Paris) 6: 407–410, 1984.

Christensen, B.V. *Collection and Cultivation of Medicinal Plants of Florida.* Florida Department of Agriculture Bulletin #14, 1950.

Clark, J.H., M.D. *A Dictionary of Practical Materia Medica.* New Delhi: 3 volumes, 1984.

Clymer, R. S., M.D. *Nature's Healing Agents.* Quakertown, PA: The Humanitarian Society, 1973.

Cook, William, M.D. *A Compend of the Newer Materia Medica.* Chicago: William Cook, 1896.

Crellin, J., and Philpott, J. *Herbal Medicine Past and Present,* vol. 2. Durham, NC: Duke University Press, 1990.

Duke, J.A. Ph.D. *CRC Handbook of Medicinal Herbs.* Boca Raton, FL: CRC Press, 1989.

Duvia et al. "Advances in the Phytotherapy of Prostatic Hypertrophy." *Med. Praxis* 4: 143–8, 1983.

Ellingwood, F. *American Materia Medica, Therapeutics and Pharmacognosy.* Evanston, IL: Ellingwoods Therapeutist, 1919.

Felter, H.W., M.D. *Eclectic Materia Medica, Pharmacology and Therapeutics.* Cincinnati, OH: John K. Scudder, 1922.

Felter, H.W., M.D. and Lloyd, J.U. *Kings American Dispensatory.* 18th ed. Cincinnati, OH: 1900.

Fyfe, J.W., M.D. *Specific Diagnosis and Specific Medication.* Cincinnati, OH: Scudder Brothers, 1909.

Geller, J. et al. "Genistein Inhibits the Growth of Human Patient BPH and Prostate Cancer in Histoculture." *Prostate* 34:75–79, 1998.

Green, J. *The Male Herbal.* Freedom, CA: The Crossing Press, 1991.

Grieve, M. *A Modern Herbal.* New York, NY: Hafner Publishing Company, 1967.

Grime, E. *Ethnobotany of the Black Americans.* Algonac, MI: Reference Publishing, 1979.

Hale, E.M., M.D. *Saw Palmetto: Its History, Botany, Chemistry, Pharmacology, Provings, Clinical Experience and Therapeutic Applications.* Philadelphia: Boericke and Tafel, 1898.

Holt, S., M.D. *Soya for Health: The Definitive Medical Guide.* Larchmont, NY: Mary Ann Liebert Publishers, 1996.

Jones, E., M.D. *Definite Medication.* Boston: Therapeutic Publishing Company, 1911.

Kikutani, T. *Combined Use of Western Therapies and Chinese Medicine.* Long Beach, CA: OH, 1987.

Kinsella, J., ed. *Seafoods and Fish Oils in Human Health and Disease.* New York: Marcel Dekker, Inc., 1987.

Kloss, J. *Back to Eden.* Washington, DC: By Author, 1939.

Kobayashi, N. et al. "Effect of Leaves of Ginkgo biloba on Hair Regrowth in C3H Strain Mice." *Yakugaku Zasshi* 113: 718–724, 1993.

Krochmal, A. and C. *A Guide to the Medicinal Plants of the United States.* New York: Quadrangle, 1973.

Leung, A.Y., Ph.D., and Foster, S. *Encyclopedia of Common Natural Ingredients Used in Food, Drugs and Cosmetics,* 2nd ed. New York: Wiley Interscience, 1996.

Lloyd, J.U. *The Origin and History of the Pharmacopoeal Drugs.* Cincinnati, Caxton Press, 1921.

Lyle, J.T., M.D. *Physio-Medical Therapeutics, Materia Medica and Pharmacy.* Salem, OH: J.M. Lyle and Brothers, 1897.

Madaus, G. *Lehrbuch der Biologischen Heilmittel.* Three volumes. Hildesheim: Georg Olms Verlag, 1979.

Marandola, P. et al. "Main Phytoderivitives in the Management of Benign Prostatic Hyperplasia." *Fitoterapia,* 68(3): 1997.

McIntyre, A. *The Complete Woman's Herbal.* New York: Henry Holt Company, 1995.

Moore, M. *Medicinal Plants of the Pacific West.* Santa Fe: Red Crane Publishers, 1993.

Morton, J.F. *Atlas of Medicinal Plants of Middle America.* Springfield, IL: Charles C. Thomas, 1981.

Morton, J.F. *500 Plants of South Florida.* Miami: E. A. Seaman, 1974.

Morton, J. F. *Wild Plants for Survival in South Florida.* Miami: Fairchild Tropical Garden, 1982.

Orbell, H. *Health from Herbs Magazine and the Medical Herbalist.* National Institute of Medical Herbalists, 1(3): 1951.

Pengelly, A. *The Constituents of Medicinal Plants.* Muswellbrook, Australia: Sunflower Herbals, 1996.

Peterson, L.A. *A Field Guide to Edible Wild Plants.* Boston: Houghton Mifflin Co., 1977.

Shamsuddin, A., M.D. "IP6 — Novel Anti-Cancer Agent." *Life Sciences* 1997, vol. 61, 343–354.

Scudder, J.M., M.D., ed. *Eclectic Medical Journal,* vol. 51. Cincinnati, OH: 1891.

Scudder, J.M., M.D., ed. *Eclectic Medical Journal,* vol. 52. Cincinnati, OH: 1892.

Shoemaker, J.V., M.D. *Materia Medica and Therapeutics.* Two volumes. Philadelphia: F.A. Davis, 1891.

Steinmetz, E.F. *Materia Medica Vegetabilis*. Two volumes. Amsterdam: self-published, 1954.

Sturtevant, W. *The Mikasuki Seminole: Medical Beliefs and Practices*. Yale University Ph.D. Thesis, 1954.

Tommi, G. et al. "Constituents of the Lipophilic Extract of the Fruits of Serenoa Repens (Bart.) small." *Gazzetta Chimica Italiana* 118:1988 823–826.

Touchstone, S.J. *Herbal & Folk Medicine of Louisiana*. Princeton, LA: Folklife Books, 1983.

Treben, Maria. *Health Through God's Pharmacy*. Steyr, Austria: Wilhelm Ennsthaler, 1984.

Vahlensieck et al. "Benign Prostatic Hyperplasia: Treatment with Sabal Fruit Extract." *Fortschritte Med* 111: 323–6, 1993.

Vogel, V.J. *American Indian Medicine*. Norman, OK: University of Oklahoma Press, 1982.

Wagner, H., and Proksch, A. *Immunostimulatory Drugs of Fungi & Higher Plants, Economic and Medicinal Plant Research*. London: Academic Press, Vol. 1, 1985.

Webster, H.J., M.D. *Dynamical Therapeutics*. San Francisco: H. J. Webster, 1898.

Weiss, R. F., M.D. *Herbal Medicine*. Gothenburg, Sweden: Beaconsfield Publications, 1988.

Werbach, M., M.D. *Nutritional Influences on Illness*. New Canaan, CT: Keats Publishing, 1988.

Whitford, A.C. *Textile Fibers Used in Eastern Aboriginal North America*. American Museum of Natural History, Anthropology Papers, vol. 38, Part I, 1941.

Williamson, E. and F. Evens. *Potters New Cyclopaedia of Botanical Drugs & Preparations*. Saffron Walden, Great Britain: C. W. Daniel Co. Ltd., 1988.

Wilt, T. et al. "Saw Palmetto Extracts for Treatment of Benign Prostatic Hyperplasia." *Journal of the American Medical Association* 280(18): 1604–9, 1998.

Yan, L. et al. "Dietary Flaxseed Supplementation and Experimental Metastasis of Melanoma Cells in Mice." *Cancer Letters* 124:181–186, 1998.

SOURCES OF SAW PALMETTO

Bulk Herbs

High-quality health food stores today carry a wide selections of herbs and natural products, and herb shops can be found almost everywhere. However, if there are no local sources of saw palmetto in your area, try any of these mail-order suppliers.

Abby's Herb Company
P.O. Box 2157
Nederland, TX 77627
888-990-HERB (4372)
Fax 409-722-2364
Web site: www.abbysherbs.com

Avena Botanicals
219 Mill Street
Rockport, ME 04856
207-594-0694

Blessed Herbs
109 Barre Plains Road
Oakham, MA 01068
800-489-4372

Dry Creek Herb Farm
13935 Dry Creek Road
Auburn, CA 95602
530-8782441

Frontier Co-op Herbs
Box 229
Norway, IA 52318
319-227-7991

Jean's Greens
R.R. 1, Box 55J
Hale Road
Rensselaerville, NY 12147
888-845-8327

Mountain Rose Herbs
20818 High Street
North San Juan, CA 95960
800-879-3337
Fax 916-292-9138

Plantation Medicinals
P.O. Box 128
Felda, FL 33930
941-675-2984
The largest commercial supplier of saw palmetto in the world.

Sage Woman Herbs
406 South 8th Street
Colorado Springs, CO 80904
888-350-3911

Tinctures

Herbalist & Alchemist, Inc.
P.O. Box 553
Broadway, NJ 08808
908-689-9020
800-611-8235 *(orders only)*

HerbPharm
Box 116
Williams, OR 97544
541-846-6262

Capsules (Ground Herbs, Sprayed Dried Extracts)

Capsules are available from many widely distributed companies, including **Rainbow Light, Zand, Solaray,** and **Nature's Way.**

Standardized Products

Available in most health food stores and pharmacies. Most contain products made by European manufacturers such as Indena (Prostaserene), Pierre Fabre Medicament (Permixon), and Pharma Stroschein GmbH (IDS 89). Bio-Botanica is an American supplier of a standardized extract (Sabaltone).

More Information on Saw Palmetto

The tapes, workbook, and proceedings of the 1998 International Saw Palmetto Symposium (August 20–22) are available through the American Herbal Products Association, 8484 Georgia Avenue, Suite 370, Silver Springs, MD, 20910, phone 301-588-1174.

WHERE TO FIND A COMPETENT HERBALIST

The American Herbalists Guild was founded in 1989 by 30 prominent American herbalists. The guild is the only organization in the United States that represents clinical or medical herbalists. Professional membership is by peer review. Members adhere to a professional code of conduct and represent some of the finest herbal practitioners in this country. The Guild also publishes a journal, *The Herbalist.*

American Herbalists Guild (AHG)
P.O. Box 70
Roosevelt, UT 84066
435-722-8434
Fax 435-722-8452
Web site: www.healthy.net/herbalists
E-mail: ahgoffice@earthlink.net

HERBAL ORGANIZATIONS

NorthEast Herbal Association (NEHA)
P.O. Box 10
Newport, NY 13416
315-845-6060
A regional organization for people who enjoy using, growing and learning about herbs. They publish a wonderful newsletter/journal.

United Plant Savers (UPS)
P.O. Box 420
East Barre, VT 05649
802-479-9825
Fax 802-476-3722
E-mail: info@www.plantsavers.org
Web site: www.plantsavers.org
*A nonprofit education organization dedicated to preserving native medicinal plants, they publish **United Plant Savers Newsletter.***

Herb Growing and Marketing
P.O. Box 245
Silver Spring, PA 17575
717-393-3295
Fax 717-393-9261
Web site: www.herbnet.com
*Publishes the **Herbal Green Pages,** is a unique resource directory of herb manufacturers, growers, stores, etc.*

Herb Research Foundation (HRF)
107 Pearl St., Suite 200
Boulder, CO 80302
303-449-2265
Web site: www.herbs.org
The HRF is a nonprofit organization that provides consumers, media, and practitioners with documented, unbiased information on herbs and their use.

HERBAL JOURNALS

HerbalGram
P.O. Box 144345
Austin, TX 78714-4345
512-926-4900
Web site: www.herbalgram.org

Herbs For Health
P.O. Box 7708
Red Oak, IA 51591-0708
Web site: www.discoverherbs.com

American Herb Association Newsletter
P.O. Box 1673
Nevada City, CA 95959

Medical Herbalism
P.O. Box 20512
Boulder, CO 80308
Web site: www.medherb.com

HERBS ELECTRONIC: GOOD RESOURCES ON THE WORLD WIDE WEB

Agricultural Research Service
www.ars-grin.gov/duke/
Dr. Jim Duke's phytochemical and ethnobotanical databases. For the serious herbalist!

Algy's Herb Page
www.algy.com/herb/index.html
Comprehensive index and archive of herb information.

American Botanical Council
www.herbalgram.org
A great assortment of information about herbs, with an especially nice introduction for beginners.

American Herbalists Guild
www.healthy.com/herbalists
Information on the AHG, a referral list to its members, education and research opportunities, and many good links.

American Herbal Pharmacopoeia™
www.herbal-ahp.org
An organization whose mission is to disseminate authoritative information regarding the proper manufacture and use of herbal medicines. Monographs are available.

Henriette's Herbal Homepage
metalab.unc.edu/herbmed
An eclectic assortment of good herb information with many good links.

The Herb Growing & Marketing Network
www.herbnet.com
Contains information on just about everything related to herbs and is updated regularly.

Herb Research Foundation
www.herbs.org
Good reviews of the most recent research in herbal medicine. Offers many good links.

A Modern Herbal
www.botanical.com/botanical/mgmh/mgmh.html
Offers the complete and searchable text of A Modern Herbal, *the classic text written by Mrs. Maude Grieve and published in 1931.*

The National Institute of Medical Herbalists
www.btinternet.com/~nimh
A basic introduction to medical herbalism and good information about the NIMH.

Southwest School of Herbal Medicine
chili.rt66.com/hrbmoore/HOMEPAGE
Michael Moore's homepage. Includes great information on herbs and education plus plant images.

Planet Herbs
www.planetherbs.com
Michael Tierra's home page. Includes an herbal studies chat room and ever-changing special features.

Medical Herbalism Homepage
medherb.com
Homepage of the quarterly journal Medical Herbalism. *Offers a free electronic subscription plus discussion of many topics relevant to clinical herbalism.*

HealthWorld Online
www.healthworld.com
Click your way through alternative medicine and you'll soon find yourself at David Hoffman's herbal materia medica (the direct route is www.healthy.net/clinic/therapy/herbal/index.html), a great breakdown of information (constituents, uses, and more) for an incredible number of herbs.

United Plant Savers
www.plantsavers.org
A nonprofit organization dedicated to preserving native medicinal plants. Web site offers an introduction to UPS, an electronic version of their newsletter, an "at-risk" list of medicinal plants, and information on upcoming events and conferences.

INDEX

Bold type indicates recipe name

OTHER STOREY TITLES YOU WILL ENJOY

Body Care Just for Men, by Jim Long. Offers dozens of health and grooming tips for skin protection, sore muscle relief, aftershaves, tonics, and more. Includes simple herbal treatments for common ailments such as sprains, cuts, abrasions, athlete's foot, jock itch, and oily/dry hair. 144 pages. Paperback. ISBN 1-58017-183-4.

Dandelion Medicine, by Brigitte Mars. This much-maligned weed is in truth one of the safest and most effective medicinal herbs available, with the power to fight infection, relieve congestion, aid digestion, and boost the immune system. Learn how to use this common plant in both food and home remedies. 128 pages. Paperback. ISBN 1-58017-207-5.

Herbal Antibiotics, by Stephen Harrod Buhner. Also in Storey's Medicinal Herb Guide series, this book presents the reader with all the current information about antibiotic-resistant microbes and the herbs that are most effective in fighting them. Readers will also find detailed, step-by-step instructions for making and using herbal infusions, tinctures, teas, and salves to treat various types of infections. 144 pages. Paperback. ISBN 1-58017-148-6.

The Herbal Home Remedy Book, by Joyce A. Wardwell. In this guide, readers will discover how to use 25 common herbs to make simple herbal remedies. Native American legends and folklore are spread throughout the book. 176 pages. Paperback. ISBN 1-58017-016-1.

Natural First Aid: Herbal Treatments for Ailments and Injuries; Emergency Preparedness; Wilderness Safety, by Brigitte Mars. Also in Storey's Medicinal Herb Guide series, this book offers quick, effective, and natural first aid suggestions for everything from ant bites to wounds. Include recipes for simple home remedies and recommends for a stocking a first aid kit for home or travel. 144 pages. Paperback. ISBN 1-58017-147-8.

Rosemary Gladstar's Herbs for Men's Health, by Rosemary Gladstar. Natural solutions to health problems common to men such as low energy, infertility, prostate problems, heart disease, hypertension, and depression. Also includes a dosage chart and extensive profiles of the most useful herbs for enhancing men's health. 80 pages. Paperback. ISBN 1-58017-151-6.

These books and other Storey Books are available at your bookstore, farm store, garden center, or directly from Storey Books, Schoolhouse Road, Pownal, Vermont 05261, or by calling 1-800-441-5700. Or visit our Web site at www.storey.com.